TALKING ABOUT APHASIA

JR
JOSEPH
ROWNTREE
FOUNDATION

The **Joseph Rowntree Foundation** has supported this project as part of its programme of research and innovative developments projects, which it hopes will be of value to policy makers and practitioners. The facts presented and views expressed in this report, however, are those of the authors and not necessarily those of the Foundation.

TALKING ABOUT APHASIA

Living with loss of language after stroke

Susie Parr, Sally Byng and *Sue Gilpin*
with **Chris Ireland**

Open University Press
Buckingham · Philadelphia

Open University Press
Celtic Court
22 Ballmoor
Buckingham
MK18 1XW

and
1900 Frost Road, Suite 101
Bristol, PA 19007, USA

First Published 1997

A catalogue record of this book is available from the British Library

ISBN   0 335 19936 4 (pb)   0 335 19937 2 (hb)

Library of Congress Cataloging-in-Publication Data
Parr, Susie, 1953–
    Talking about aphasia: living with loss of language after stroke
    / Susie Parr, Sally Byng, and Sue Gilpin; with Chris Ireland.
        p.   cm.
    Includes bibliographical references (p.   ).
    ISBN 0-335-19937-2 (hb.) – ISBN 0-335-19936-4 (pb)
    1. Aphasia.   2. Aphasia – Case studies.   3. Cerebrovascular
disease – Complications.   I. Byng, Sally, 1956–   II. Gilpin,
Sue.   III. Ireland, Chris.   IV. Title.
    RC425.P376   1997
362.1'968552–dc21   97–15402
                                                                              CIP

Typeset by Type Study, Scarborough
Printed in Great Britain by Biddles Ltd, Guildford and King's Lynn

Contents

Notes on the authors

Susie Parr has worked as a speech and language therapist in Ireland, Liverpool and Bristol and has undertaken research into the impact of aphasia upon literacy practices. She is currently Research Fellow in the Department of Clinical Communication Studies, City University, London.

Sally Byng is Professor of Communication Disability in the Department of Clinical Communication Studies, City University. She trained as a speech and language therapist and has written on a number of topics associated with aphasia, including language processing and outcomes measurement.

Sue Gilpin was working as a Head of a Language Faculty in a large comprehensive school when she had a stroke and became aphasic in 1987. Since that time, she has gained an MA in special education. She is a member of the Council of Action for Dysphasic Adults.

Chris Ireland is a teacher and a trained counsellor. Since her stroke in 1988, which left her with aphasia, she has worked on a research project investigating the value of counselling for aphasic people, and has written, lectured and run workshops on different aspects of aphasia.

Foreword
by *Chris Ireland*

This is a collective of voices, often to be not listened to and often not heard and often not to understand. This is a very readable book — filter from complex to be so easily to read. Each chapter invites the reader to the world-word-lives of people with aphasia. Each title of each chapter show the flexible, empathetic, powerful medium of language — reading and out-pick out issues, when the reader ready to dialogues.

This book belong to the people who tell their stories. Also it belongs with you — the readers to reflect their own experiences and learn and share various perceptions. Living with aphasia is facing daily struggle — pain, confusions, isolating, anxiety — and learning and understanding within the social world — so noisy, so stressful, so dirty polluted, needy, greedy. But some care, some are open to learn and some have vision.

Also it belonged to those who worked very hard, using their talents, learning about pain and limitations from others. In feedback and empowering people to tell their stories, to filter, open hole the stony wall, graphical, strongly, powerful. Not only to reflect but also to suggest more clear and helpful advisory support. Also, with the disability movement, towards more understanding and collective voice to campaign for better services for each needs.

Readership of this book — some will more understanding — some with fired and encouraged with the fight and seek support. Anothers will learn more about the complexity in the struggles of people with aphasia — both social issues and warring impairments. Illness and disability are worsened depends on others reactions, or help or not — understanding and care — real care and reflect on more humane social policies and advocate for invisible disabilities to become more visible.

Preface

This book is about the experience of losing language as a result of a stroke. It is based on the accounts of fifty aphasic people who took part in a research project, run between 1994 and 1996 in the Department of Clinical Communication Studies, City University, London. The project was funded by the Joseph Rowntree Foundation. The respondents agreed to take part in in-depth interviews in which they talked about their experience of aphasia, its impact on their lives, their hopes for the future, the obstacles they face, and the support available to them. The focus falls exclusively on the views and experiences of aphasic people themselves, not those of their friends and family, nor those of the various professional groups whom they have encountered. We make no apology for maintaining this perspective throughout the book. Losing language can mean that others start to take over, with the result that people with aphasia are often side-lined.

This is the first time that an extensive account of aphasia, given by those who have first-hand knowledge of it, is delivered on its own terms and not placed in the context of professional, clinical, medical or academic concerns. As such, it can claim to break new ground. Although issues relating to the delivery of therapeutic services and the medical and linguistic aspects of aphasia have been studied in some detail, the long-term consequences and the significance of aphasia for those who have it have never been investigated in any sustained and systematic way. Similarly, while we acknowledge the importance of the views and experiences of the friends and family of aphasic people, these were not addressed in the project, precisely because we wanted the accounts of aphasic people themselves to be heard.

In the book, we try to convey the experience of what it is like to live with aphasia. In Chapters 1 and 2, aphasic people give accounts of having a stroke, impressions of hospital and describe their first perceptions of their language impairment. They describe early treatments and services and the ups and downs of returning home. Chapter 3 explores the impact of aphasia, in the long-term, on the work, education and leisure opportunities of aphasic people. The impact of aphasia on personal relationships with family and friends is described in Chapter 4. Chapter 5 maps out the long-term, changing needs of aphasic people and examines how successfully these are met by health, social care and other services at different points in time. Chapter 6 draws together several accounts in exploring the changing needs of aphasic people regarding the content, timing and presentation of information. Ways in which people understand their aphasia and the different ways of coping with it are explored in Chapter 7. Chapter 8 asks in what ways, and on whose terms, aphasia can be described as a disability. The final chapter trawls the many different accounts of aphasia to draw out principles for learning to live with the loss of language. A detailed account of how the study was carried out is given in the Appendix. Readers interested in exploring some issues in more depth will find a list of relevant texts in the Further Reading section.

Three main themes recur throughout the book. First, as far as possible the difficulties encountered by aphasic people are depicted, not as inevitable consequences of the impairment itself, but as obstacles which might be removed with appropriate action and support. Secondly, various resources and services are described and evaluated only in so far as they impinge, or fail to do so, on the lived experience of people who have aphasia. Thirdly, the accounts given by aphasic people allow a detailed and sustained exploration of the intricate nature of language. Throughout the book, we return again and again to the importance of language, in maintaining relationships, in negotiating and controlling the help that is given, and in understanding and coping with a suddenly acquired, long-term impairment.

The book has been written with a number of different audiences in mind. Most importantly, we hope that aphasic people, their families and friends will be attracted to it and find it helpful to learn about how others have dealt with aphasia. It is for this reason that, although it is informed by current theories and debates, the book has not been produced as an academic text. As far as possible, it has been written in straightforward and accessible language and it is unreferenced.

In addition, we hope that those who provide nursing, medical and rehabilitation services to people with aphasia, together with those involved in community and social care services will find it useful to read about what it is like to have aphasia and to learn about the many areas of unmet need. We hope that those responsible for planning health and social care services for aphasic people will read it, and that it will be useful to those who provide information. Those working within voluntary and charitable organisations which offer support to aphasic people should find that the book raises a number of issues which are relevant to their services. Finally, we hope that the book will be of special interest to speech and language therapists, as we think it offers a new and challenging perspective on aphasia.

At this point, we wish to acknowledge all those who have made this book possible. First, we would like to thank the Joseph Rowntree Foundation for funding the project and for their sustained support through all its ups and downs. We owe an enormous debt of thanks to Jane Ritchie, of Social and Community Planning Research, who acted as consultant to the project. She was instrumental in shaping the design of the project and in setting high standards for the research. At every stage, we have benefited from her understanding, both of the issues and of the process of investigation, and her clarity of thought. Kit Ward, also of Social and Community Planning Research, offered skilled and sensitive help in training our interviewing skills and in undertaking some interviews herself.

Throughout the project, we have benefited from the input of two advisory groups. We would like to acknowledge the contribution of Sally French, David Ellis, Margot Larkin, Sheila Wirz, Mike Bury and Judith Waterman, all of whom offered consistent interest and support and who managed to focus their diverse professional concerns into constructive and useful advice. The other advisory group was made up of people who have first-hand experience of aphasia. Harry Clarke, Sue Boazman, Lynn Thomson, Graham Kellie, Trevor Walker, Jasvinder Khosa and Anna Ashworth contributed to an invaluable, on-going commentary which has enriched every stage of the project. We would all like to thank Carole Pound. From the start, she has proved an unstinting source of humour, creative ideas, practical help and encouragement. We would also like to acknowledge the personal support offered by Martin and Ellen Parr, Winifred and Douglas Mitchell, David Kessler, Liz Lee, Matthew, Gabriel and Laura Byng, Jackie Strong, Denise Norman-Dent, Carole Watkins, Sue Neale, Ralph and Sylvia Gilpin, David Bennett, Ralph Norbury, Sally Inman and Magdlin Babiker.

Finally, and most importantly, we would like to thank all the people who took part in the project and who talked about the experience of aphasia with such thoughtfulness and honesty. We hope we have done justice to their accounts.

1

What is aphasia?

Aphasia: some facts

- Aphasia is a language impairment. It can affect many aspects of communication including speech, writing, reading, gesture and understanding of the spoken word.
- Aphasia is caused when certain areas of the brain become damaged. These areas control language, just as other areas of the brain control movement and co-ordination. In most people, the areas which control language are found in the front region of the left-hand side of the brain.
- The commonest cause of aphasia is stroke. About a third of all people who have strokes develop aphasia. Other causes of aphasia include head injury and tumours.
- In the United Kingdom, at least 20,000 people become aphasic every year.

'My mind is one hundred per cent . . . um . . . all the time. Speaking is bad.'
Sharon

'The trouble me that talking . . . list . . . listening and talking can't speak. Can't speak you know. Explaining things. Oh . . . that's problem. But trouble was I know expl . . . which like this, like was me. I know, remember so and so. Yeah. Leap, leap. And . . . and remember the words, I tripping up in words really. Tripping up in words. What's the name of so and so?'
Roger

'No I can't write now. Oh, me name, that's all. I can write er . . . odd words but I couldn't write . . . I can't spell so to write to wri . . . well . . . eh . . . eh . . . I wrote a letter the other day. I had my kitchen done and wrote what I thought was a letter to the . . . um . . . When I come home he said: "I'm ever so sorry. I couldn't understand this. Could you explain it to me what it was?" Er . . . I said: "Can't you?" "No", he said, "I can't understand that." And I looked at it and it were a load of rubbish.'

Pearl

'They were talking to me and sometimes I didn't even know . . . they'd say something but by the end of the sentence they was saying I didn't know what it was because I'm still thinking of the first little bit. It was . . . that was strange, you know, because I really wanted to get into people's conversations but I couldn't . . . and I would look at them.'

Jenny

'Sometime to make sentences or read sentences hard, hard. But you can repeat word. I think you can more or less you can understand what is written. I think so, if not hard words . . . simple words, not big words.'

Govi

Interviewer:	*What happened when you tried to say something?*
Jack:	*No, no*
Interviewer:	*Nothing?*
Jack:	*No*
Interviewer:	*Mm. Can you remember what that felt like?*
Jack:	*Ooooh . . . buh*
Interviewer:	*Frustrating? You look very frustrated*
Jack:	*Yeah . . . ooooh*
Interviewer:	*And angry?*
Jack:	*Yeah*

Sharon, Roger, Pearl, Jenny, Govi and Jack are talking about an experience which is hard for many people to imagine or understand: the loss of language. They have 'aphasia'. It is perhaps hard to understand what aphasia is because few people think about how they communicate and use language, just as those who are able to do so may give little thought to their ability to walk, pick up a book or drink a cup of tea. Families may enjoy observing and helping young children as they try to communicate before they can talk, as they develop speech and understanding and as they learn to read and write. This may be one of the few times that language and communication are consciously considered. Often, they are not thought about at all, especially if the child has no problems along the way. People may have little awareness of the many ways in which they communicate, and think that language is nothing more than the ability to speak and hear. By taking away or damaging language, aphasia reveals the complexity and skill of communication, how many forms it can take, and how vital it is. So what exactly is aphasia?

What is aphasia?

- Aphasia can affect different aspects of language:
  - ability to put ideas and intentions into spoken and written language;
  - ability to spell;
  - ability to put words together in grammatical sentences;
  - ability to understand what is said;
  - ability to understand the written word;
  - ability to understand and use other forms of communication, for example gesture.
- Aphasia can take different forms.
- Aphasia can vary in severity.
- Aphasia can change over time.
- Aphasia does not affect intelligence.

Aphasia affects different aspects of language

The extracts from interviews with Roger, Pearl, Jack and Govi show how, for some people, the capacity to speak is affected by aphasia. Roger speaks in very short phrases, has difficulty finding the words he wants to express his thoughts and, as he says, *'explaining things'*. The sentences he says don't always sound correct, and this is because he has trouble with grammar and organising the ways words can go together. When he says: *'Leap. Leap.'* he is referring to the way in which he has to struggle to keep to his point. His mind is leaping around.

Jack's spoken language is very impaired. Although he can use the words *'yes'* and *'no'*, and can say some short phrases, Jack has to communicate what he feels largely through his facial expression, his gestures and the tone of his voice.

Govi and Pearl make the point that aphasia affects other aspects of communication as well as speech. Reading and writing are just as much communication skills as talking and listening, and they, too, can be impaired by aphasia. Pearl's account of leaving instructions for a builder illustrates how people with aphasia may find themselves unable to write what they want. Aphasia may affect the ability to produce writing, to use grammatically correct sentences, and to spell. Reading can also become difficult. For example, Govi can only read text which is clear and simply expressed.

But it is Jenny who talks about the aspect of aphasia which is in some ways the least obvious: it can affect a person's ability to follow what is being said. The aphasic person can hear others talking, but may find it difficult to understand what is being said. Many aphasic people find this becomes worse when they are tired, or when there is too much going on around them and they are having to deal with a lot of background noise. The difficulty in understanding language is nothing to do with hearing loss. The language can be heard but not understood.

In order to appreciate what this must be like, it is helpful to think about trying to communicate using a foreign language. Vocabulary and grammatical patterns have to be learnt and practised. In addition, the learner has to try to understand what is being said. This process is helped if native speakers talk slowly, simplify their language, repeat what they have said and back it up with gestures and drawings. Noisy or distracting environments can make it difficult to follow someone who is speaking in a different language. The whole process of trying to understand what is said or trying to say something demands concentrated effort and can be tiring. This is also the case with aphasia. Many aphasic people find that they have to work hard at following and taking part in a conversation. Sometimes they need to ask the person with whom they are talking to repeat what has been said and to talk slowly. Often, people with aphasia need to cut out background noise and other distractions so that they can concentrate on communication. The effort that is needed can often increase levels of fatigue and stress with the result that communication becomes more difficult.

Aphasia can take different forms

Not everyone has the same kind of aphasia. It can manifest itself in many different ways. Thus, some aphasic people like Roger and Govi have difficulty piecing words together into sentences. Roger cuts out some small grammatical words like 'the' and 'is' which are generally used to hold sentences together. He uses the important or 'key' words to convey his meaning. In contrast, Pearl does not appear to have a problem with making grammatical sentences. However, her speech is hesitant and she can lose track of what she is saying especially when she can't think of the word she wants: '. . .wrote what I thought was a letter to the . . . um . . .'. Others who have aphasia may find that, instead of their speech being slow and hesitant, and coming out in short phrases, they speak very fluently and indeed have trouble controlling the outpouring of speech. People who have 'fluent aphasia' can find that it is difficult to be specific. They may struggle to answer questions or give precise information.

Aphasia can vary in severity

As well as taking different forms, aphasia can vary in severity. For some people, like Jenny, aphasia means they have occasional difficulty finding a word they want to use, and perhaps some problems reading or writing complicated material. For others, aphasia impairs the ability to understand what is said, makes even the simplest writing incomprehensible and reduces them to silence or to a few phrases which they use over and over again. The very fact that aphasia can affect so many different aspects of language, and to such varying degrees makes it more difficult to understand and explain. Aphasia is not straightforward or simple.

Aphasia can change over time

Aphasia can change as time passes. Some language can return in the days, weeks and months following the stroke, and speech and language therapy can be very effective in helping to bring back skills which seemed to be lost. It is also possible to get used to aphasia, to disguise it, and to find ways of dealing with it. Nevertheless, many people find that, in the long run, their aphasia does not disappear as they had hoped. It is there for good, and they, their family and friends are faced with the task of learning to live with an impairment that affects every aspect of their lives.

Intelligence is not affected by aphasia

Sharon expresses a crucial point about people with aphasia when she says: '*My mind is one hundred per cent . . . speaking is bad.*' This refers to the fact that the person with aphasia is able to think, feel, remember and plan, even though their language is not working. Aphasia damages the lines of communication going in and out, not the thought, intelligence and experience of the person. Again, this is hard to grasp, especially in a society that places value on the ability to communicate through speech and writing, and indeed which considers these skills to be signs of intelligence.

In the interviews upon which this book is based, many of these features of aphasia are illustrated. Some of the people interviewed are able to talk very fluently, with perhaps only the occasional hesitation or difficulty in finding the word they want. Some people talk copiously, and find it difficult to make their point concisely. Some struggle to put together a sentence. Others can use only one or two words and have to rely on using their tone of voice, gestures and facial expression to communicate what they want to say. In the quotations used in this book, hesitations which occur in the person's speech are indicated by dots (. . .). If a sentence or a block of speech has been left out because it is not relevant to the point, this is indicated by a dash (—). In some cases, it is necessary to reproduce the interviewer's questions, so that the answers may be understood.

Who gets aphasia?

While older people are more likely to have strokes and develop aphasia, young people and even children can also be affected. Although stroke has not been linked with any particular socio-economic group, members of some cultures (for example, people of Southern Asian origin) are more vulnerable to diabetes, heart disease and other problems that are linked with stroke. Men are slightly more at risk of stroke than women. But stroke and aphasia can affect people of any age, and background as the following accounts show.

Betty is 76, widowed and lives alone in Manchester. Having worked as an office manager, she retired and concentrated on her interest in writing articles and stories and started an Open University philosophy course. She had a stroke ten years ago. Describing herself before she became aphasic, she says: *'I always knew I was a know-all —. I used to understand everything er . . . and at the end of it I could sort of say a sentence which would sort of wrap it up if you know what I mean. I just thinking Sir Thomas Aquinas he said: "I thank God that I have understood every word that I read." In a very small way I used to be like that. Writing and talking used to be my thing. I've talked all the night and it was enjoyable to me as, well, chocolates and cinnamon to anybody else. That was the way I lived.'*

Cath is 47, married and has two children in their twenties. She was working as a hotel manager, in a very isolated location, when she had a stroke. Describing what she was like before she became aphasic, she points out how she was able to deal with the demands of her job, and her college training: *'Manager and College and enormous words and writing and reading and understand letters and I can't now.'*

Kiran is 37, married and lives in Birmingham. He was working as a senior teacher when he had a brain haemorrhage which left him with aphasia. He describes himself before his stroke as *'garrulous'*, someone who loved humour and could switch easily between languages: *'. . . our humour would play Panjabi-English'* . . ., but also as someone who took his work very seriously: '*I had written a few articles on education. And language was very, very important to me.*' Kiran's love of humour, company and language developed during his childhood in Northern Ireland: '*Now in, where I was born, it's an area of writers. So humour is particularly important, even now — I'm interested in literature — I come from a Catholic town and I'm not used to being alone for any length of time.*'

Fred is 61 and lives with his wife in Liverpool. He was 41, working as a railway shunter and his two children were about to leave school when he had a stroke. Talking about what he was like before he had aphasia he says: '*I used to be able to spell 'precocious' but I can't . . . I used to love reading . . . books. I still can't concentrate on books, mind. I read papers but not books. I used to love . . . read . . . oh piles and piles of books . . .*'

These examples bring home the fact that aphasia can happen to anybody. It interrupts lives busy with work, interests and relationships. People who become aphasic have histories which do not disappear when language departs. One of the many challenges they face involves finding connections between the new 'aphasic self' and the person who perhaps used to enjoy chatting to friends or reading novels, whose work involved writing, speaking and listening or whose quickfire, witty coments would make people laugh. In this book, we hope to explore how aphasia can change many aspects of peoples' lives, the barriers they face, and the ways in which they cope.

The onset of aphasia

Coming from different backgrounds, locations, cultures and support systems, the people we interviewed spoke about aphasia from many different points of view and about various ways of dealing with it. But despite their differences, and despite the fact that they were talking about events which had taken place years before, everyone was able to describe the alarming experience of having a stroke in some detail and to convey the drama and shock of those first moments. For some, this involved sudden collapse and loss of consciousness, as Lionel, a former priest, explains:

*'I . . . filed in with priests and things and . . . suddenly I thought this is funny . . .
um . . . that's not right and I get . . . got up and went to the door and you know
that . . . I don't know I fell down and that's it. I can't remember anything at all.'*

In some cases, the aphasic person's partner was the first one to discover
that something was wrong:

*'Drive home . . . watching the news, putting the stuff for food, you know, and
about eleven o'clock ah well, we'll go upstairs and sleep. Now in the morning my
wife made a cup of tea . . . 8 o'clock . . . 8 o'clock, shake, shake. No answer. Dead.
Rushed to London Hospital with a drips . . .'*

Robert

*'Um . . . night-time . . . um . . . home, tired and sleepy . . . awful . . . um . . .
Sunday, Sunday and morning, shaking, she no answer.'*

Ken

A few people remained conscious for a time and are able to recall the
sensations of the stroke as it was actually happening, and even the first
signs of their aphasia:

*'All of a sudden, I became sweaty and um . . . er . . . um . . . became stuck on
"When". I said: "When . . . when . . . when . . ." Er . . . I was embarrassed for
my friends, for they had come and my invitation — and I wanted them to feel
comfortable. So, when I get stuck on "When" the more I become embarrassed, the
more I become anxious, and that's the cycle. And I'm not . . . I'm a fighter
basically. So I thought: "Damn this, I need to fight it, whatever it is." — By this
time I was all sweaty and um . . . I didn't know what was happening but I was
more concerned about my friends. My wife came down and er . . . I became, for
the first time, frightened. And I started losing . . . er . . . feeling right down my
body . . .'*

Kiran

All but one of the fifty people who took part in this study were admit-
ted to hospital when they had the stroke, and some went on to different
hospitals for treatment and rehabilitation. Length of time in hospital
varied, the shortest stay being for five days and the longest for fourteen
months. It was therefore in the hospital environment, rather than at
home, that most people started to realise that something had happened to
their language. The next chapter will begin with these early experiences
and the thoughts, feelings and fears concerning both aphasia and the
physical problems which can result from stroke.

2

'Is frightened. Is frightened': the early experience of stroke and aphasia

Emerging from the drowsiness following the stroke, reactions vary as aphasic people start to take stock of their situation. Some describe the first realisation of what has happened as a violent shock *'like falling down from a plane'*. Some recall piecing together events and feeling anxious about their future. Some were bewildered and uncertain. Some felt imprisoned, cut off or lonely. Others felt as if they had returned to babyhood, finding themselves being washed, lifted, moved, worked on by the army of nurses and therapists, and unable to speak:

'The um . . . no speech nothing . . . maybe one sentence and . . . um . . . and physical side um . . . the arm and legs um . . . first off in a wheelchair all the time . . . um . . . the um . . . physio come to see the hospital . . . the ward um . . . one, two times a day and um . . . the OT and the . . . oh . . . in the kitchens and bathroom and shower and stuff is er . . . um . . . um . . . maybe mean newborn and stuff . . .'
Sharon

These reactions, ranging from fear to amusement, from despair to enjoyment, from shock to detachment suggest that there may be no way of predicting individual responses in the first few days following a stroke. Because of the aphasia, it may be difficult for the person to communicate feelings and needs to others. As a result, those around the aphasic person may not know what kind of support to offer.

Some early reactions to stroke

- *'Is frightened. Is frightened'.*
- *'I was quite happy because I didn't know what was going on'.*
- *'Unbelievable is so awful.'*
- *'Everything been washed from my brain.'*
- *'I was completely blank.'*
- *'Dream world. I was in a daze.'*
- *'I found it funny.'*
- *'Where am I? What is happening to me?'*
- *'It was just as if I had died.'*
- *'It was like hitting somewhere at 100 miles per hour.'*
- *'Everything went over my head.'*
- *'Everyone was talking to me.'*
- *'I was stuck inside.'*
- *'I was delighted by all the attention.'*
- *'Newborn.'*
- *'Big cot. All fence . . . fenced me around'.*

'My bloody body wasn't working': the physical aftermath of stroke

Over the course of the first few days, some of the immediate physical effects of the stroke start to became apparent. As with aphasia, the severity, extent and nature of physical impairment following stroke can vary. Most people who took part in this study experienced some physical effects in the first instance. In some cases, these were limited to a sense that things were not quite right: '. . . *one of my hands don't seem to correspond to the other — And I know I feel different.'* But for others, more major physical problems quickly became obvious. These included *paralysis* or *weakness* of limbs, *loss of sensation, difficulty swallowing* and *crying.*

Paralysis, weakness and loss of sensation

The physical aftermath of stroke can include paralysis or weakness, usually down one side of the body, visual problems and numbness or a sensation of pins and needles. These can all affect a person's ability to carry out the movements involved in actions such as sitting, standing, picking things up, walking and turning round. Thus, following a stroke, it may be difficult to do ordinary things like lifting a cup to take a drink, or going to the toilet.

Difficulty swallowing

Weakness and paralysis of the muscles of the face, mouth and throat often causes difficulty swallowing following stroke. Liquids can be particularly difficult to control, and dribbling is common. The person's speech may become unclear if the muscles of the lips, tongue, throat and palate are affected. In addition, weakness of the muscles can cause one side of the face to drop, and this can make the person's appearance change.

Crying

One problem which many people encounter, especially in the early days after the stroke, is the tendency to cry uncontrollably. This seems to be a common experience and does not always mean that the person is feeling sad or upset, although of course many people can feel distressed as they start to realise what has happened. It seems that the stroke can damage the person's ability to control weeping. Tears are easily triggered, even by sympathetic comments, expressions of affection and concern, and items on TV. '. . . part of a film, if it's sad and my God, that's it.'

'How would you feel?': first reactions to physical impairment

Immediate reactions to realisations of physical impairment vary from person to person. Feelings of *shock, anger, frustration* and *distress*, are common, especially in response to major mobility problems. Many, even those who have apparently minimal physical impairments, look back at their previous abilities with feelings of *grief* and *loss*:

'Bear in mind in the first year I go to pieces because knowing I used to physical fit and all.'

Vincent

'You're perfect. You're perfect. Suddenly you're paralysed. How would you feel?'
Govi

For some, the *embarrassment* of finding themselves unable to control dribbling or crying seems as trying as the frustrations of limited mobility:

'I've been sitting here like this and all of a sudden it will start, you know, I just couldn't stop it. Tears come and watch the television and that and children or elderly or anything like that — I felt a bit shamed, you know, because crying in front of other people.'

Ted

Sometimes physical changes can lead to a sense of *lost identity*, especially when personal appearance is affected. This is particularly the case if a person's facial appearance changes as a result of muscle weakness, as Rebecca describes:

'I don't know whether it's because you sort of take on a completely new image . . . you lose your normality, don't you, when your face has dropped?'

Physical impairments following stroke can diminish with time and with the help of physical therapies. Those who experience more profound and long-lasting physical effects find that it can take a long time to grow accustomed to the changes:

'I always compare myself . . . when I in front of the mirror. I see myself as Kiran Mark One. But I'm Kiran Mark Two.'

'I . . . dumb': first realisations of aphasia

Disturbing though the immediate physical effects of the stroke are, the realisation that something has also happened to their language seems to be a harrowing experience for everybody. The loss of the ability to speak is usually obvious, as people struggle to express their thoughts although sometimes it takes time to realise the message is not getting across: *'I didn't realise. I thought I was talking properly.'* Others find themselves completely unable to speak:

'I stuck the word — No bloody speech at all.'

Robert

'Speak . . . blank . . . blank . . . start again . . . muddled.'

Ken

The difficulty in speaking seems to be particularly upsetting when it involves not being able to find important words, for example, the names of friends and family members. However, for some people, even attempting to say someone's name is out of the question because they find themselves unable to stop repeating a single word or phrase. Ken, for example, was initially only able to say the word *'Question'* over and over again, while Colin was limited to *'Bloody hell!'* and *'Let's have a party!'* Attempts to communicate through writing are often equally unsuccessful: *'My husband would say: "Try writing what you want." But I'd just write squiggles . . .'*

Attempting the usual occupations of hospital life, like ticking off choices on a menu card, looking at magazines or selecting a book from the library trolley, can bring home to some people the fact that their reading has also been affected. For Rose, this was the first indication that something quite fundamental had changed:

'I felt as though I was helpless and I couldn't get out and um . . . I say I couldn't read . . . I could not make the symbols out . . . um . . . a . . . writing. I mean, I could look at that and not read it. And that was a frightening thing to me because I mean I obviously I could read before and I mean people would keep bringing me in these Cosmopolitans *and . . . and . . . I was sort of said . . . er . . . I mean noises . . . er . . . thanks and I couldn't read them. I mean I absolutely couldn't read them.'*

'I couldn't speak what was wrong': aphasia and being ill

Anxiety and uncertainty are common reactions to illness, especially when it is sudden, dramatic and unexpected, like stroke. Usually, it is possible to tackle and, to a certain extent, contain anxiety through the use of language: asking questions, getting information about the cause and nature of the condition, understanding the prognosis, finding out what to expect in terms of time-span in hospital and treatments, and obtaining comfort and reassurance. Those who have aphasia may not be able to deal with their anxieties and uncertainties in this way. They find it difficult to ask for assistance, to find out exactly what has happened and what the outlook is, to give answers to questions from nursing and medical staff, and to express their concern. From the start, aphasia means that they can exert little control over their illness:

'I guess one day he did come round to some of the staff because . . . I don't remember . . . they er . . . the words . . . I couldn't speak, you see. No way of communicating and er . . . er . . . then he would start talking to . . . er . . . but he was talking to me . . . more quickly. I couldn't understand what he was . . . er . . . slowly, slowly, slowly.'

Uncertainty about the condition

Some people know that they have had a stroke, perhaps because they have, in the past, witnessed a friend or relative going through the same thing. However, those who don't have this experience to draw on, and who cannot take in information, may consider their symptoms and jump to the wrong conclusion. Rebecca thought *'I was going out of my head'* and for Mike it was as if *'I was bloody daft. Like a school-kid.'* Charles watched other people's reactions to him and remembers what he felt: *'I'm thinking they're thinking I've gone barmy.'*

In some cases, the impression that the problems are being caused by mental illness is strengthened by encounters with medical and therapeutic staff.

Not understanding what had happened to him and the purpose of his treatments, *Alf* found his first experience of speech and language therapy had an infuriating effect. He needed information, but didn't get it. Instead, he was launched into a series of what seemed to him bizarre and pointless activities. He started to suspect that the therapy was being used to check his mental state: *'She and I took a dislike to each other as soon as we was talking because she was trying to make me do something and I did not want to do it and I've gone: "What the hell do I want to take any notice of her for?" And she used to . . . and it was cards, we used to have cards and it is "Why is that man change gear?" and I used to say: "Well how do I know?" Slowly, slow version because I was pretty . . . not all that great in speaking, so it was relearning again the speech and I used to go: "But . . . but . . . but . . . why . . . me . . . no . . . er . . . ill?" More like pidgin-fashion and we was always arguing — What it actually was was I thought somebody was trying to make me look a dim dim. What they call that word? Illit . . . ? . . . When you can't read and write — They was trying to do something that was . . . I knew was wrong and I . . . when anybody tries to do that to me I'm the first one to beg to differ. And I thought at first they was trying to put me into an asylum.'*

Confusion about the role of professionals

Unable to ask for or understand information, many, like Alf, feel unsure of who is who among those working on their bodies and speech, and caring for them during their days in hospital. The boundaries between physiotherapists, occupational therapists, speech and language therapists, nurses, social workers may be unclear, especially for those unused to hospital culture. It is not easy to sort this out without language, as Trevor explains:

'I . . . I . . . couldn't ask them what they was. I hadn't a clue who they were sort of thing. That's the only thing that got you barmy sort of thing because I couldn't'

How aphasia affects the experience of dealing with illness

- Difficulty expressing concern and asking for information: *'I thought I was asking the doctors questions but I wasn't.'*
- Difficulty understanding what is being said: *'. . . he was talking to me quickly.'*

- Uncertainty about outlook and treatment: *'I thought it would be a week, two weeks.'*
- Uncertainty about nature of condition: *'I thought I was loolally.'*
- Confusion about role of professionals: *'I hadn't a clue who they were.'*

'Derelict': first reactions to aphasia

As they start to take in the nature and effects of their language impairment, people can react in different ways, with powerful and emotional feelings. Because of the aphasia, often it is not possible to handle these strong emotions by expressing and sharing them with others. They have to remain bottled up within the aphasic person.

Fear and anxiety

For many people, the experience of aphasia is frightening. Some fear can arise from a growing awareness of what has been lost. Some arises from uncertainty about what has happened, and about whether the condition is going to get worse. In addition, fear is often rooted in concern about the long-term prospects:

'I was desperate because I thought: "My God . . . what about my job?"'

Rebecca

'I couldn't work out how I was going to carry on'.

Christopher

Others feel anxious about immediate concerns, for example, whether or not they will be able to communicate the fact that they want to go to the toilet and whether they will wet the bed.

Anger and frustration

The frustration of not being able to communicate frequently leads to feelings of anger. Jack shakes his fist when asked about his feelings at the time and Pearl recalls:

'I was mad. I was mad in here that it wouldn't come out — When I did try to say to something um . . . and it all come out . . . well gobbledegook . . . um . . . and I knew what I was going to say but I couldn't say it and I used to get mad — Mad with myself.'

The anger and frustration may be intensified because they themselves can't be expressed and explained in words. However, they can be expressed through other means: banging on the table, crying, shouting and swearing. Les found that, while *'other words is hopeless'*, he found himself able to swear *'loud and clear.'* He noticed this in other people too. While it sometimes seems impossible for aphasic people to find the words they want, there seems to be little difficulty locating swear words. Just as they struggle to control their weeping, some people find themselves unable to stem the flow of swear words. This can be deeply embarrassing, especially for someone who rarely swore before the stroke.

Devastation

An overwhelming awareness of loss causes a sense of devastation to some people. Govi was so distressed by his aphasia he felt like giving up: *'Oh my God. I want to die — when I could not speak — Because I know I could not live that way.'*

For Betty, the loss of the language skills which had been so central to her life had a traumatic effect. This was worsened by the fact that she was unable to find out what her prospects for recovery were: *'I was absolutely devastated. I came round and realised that it was gone and nobody would tell me when it would come back . . . er . . . I suppose they didn't know.'*

Isolation

Unable to share their feelings with others because of their aphasia, some people start to feel isolated and cut off. Aphasic people use powerful images to convey the sense of isolation as they find themselves: *'cocooned in this lonely shell'* and *'stuck inside.'* The word *'derelict,'* used by Roger to describe his feelings at the time, manages to convey his feelings of devastation, loss and loneliness.

'I was telling her. I was telling her': other people and aphasia

For some people, anger can arise, not so much from the frustrations of their own attempts to communicate but in response to the way in which other people, including family members and professionals, react to their difficulties with communication. One of the commonest, and most infuriating, experiences is that of being 'talked over'. For Martha, a former doctor, this was particularly galling:

'I was furious with the nurses because . . . well two nurses came on one and another side of me and they . . . they . . . they discussed me . . . over . . . never . . .

never thought of me at all. Never. I couldn't help . . . you know I wasn't able to speak very well by that time. I was furious with, you know — I'm usually the person to do the speaking.'

Many people shared this kind of experience and describe it with anger.

Fred felt that people talking to him in hospital should have made an effort to help him use his available communication skills. Instead he was 'talked over', and felt shunned and pushed aside: *'People couldn't understand my speech at all . . . but I could still say "Yes" and "No" . . . things that could . . . People could understand me. If they could help me by speaking to me it would help me. Yes. Even the doctor would come in and ask my wife questions, not me. He would come in and ask the wife: "How are you today? How is he today?" I was sat along, silent — I kept trying to tell him: "Ask me. Ask me." But er that time they . . . they say to her: "Has he slept all night?" And I knew the answer to that. But he would ask her: "And has he been can-tankerous today?" '* Added to the frustration of this kind of experience, Fred also suffered the humiliation of not being able to get through to a nurse the fact that he needed to go to the toilet. Eighteen years after the event, telling this story still makes him upset: *'They tried to take me for a little walk down the corridor. I couldn't hardly walk at all then. I can remember this. I tried to tell the nurse I wanted to go to the toilet. But no one would . . . er . . . she kept pulling me down the corridor. I had to do it as I stood up there. Ooh . . . I remember that. It was terrible — And the nurse said to me, as I went she said . . . done it in my trousers . . . she said: "Why didn't you tell me?" And I was . . . me . . . I was* <u>telling</u> *her. I was* <u>telling</u> *her: "I want to go back to the toilet." But no-one wouldn't listen to me.'*

As well as being 'talked over', Cath had the experience of being talked down to. She describes how some of the hospital staff made her feel like a child when they made her try and ask for the things she needed:

'Angry, angry . . . hit really, but not — A girl really, a girl. "Bathroom? Eh? Eh? You bathroom? No? Or bathroom?" Or something, you know — Yeah oh and walking, you know walking. "Well, say, say, say." Well why should I?'

'You've got to do something': starting to cope

Reacting with a tumult of emotions to the uncertain and frustrating cir-cumstances in which they find themselves, many aphasic people quickly start to martial their resources in attempts to cope with what is happen-ing. In some cases, this involves drawing on their own memories and experiences and trying to talk themselves through the experience. Often, deprived of language, they are dependent on the respect and sensitivity with which they are treated by others to raise their spirits and make them feel more in control of the situation. Finding practical solutions to communication problems also helps, as does some contact with others who are going through the same thing.

Fighting talk

Starting to get over the initial shock of the stroke, some people are able to use 'fighting talk' to summon up their will-power and determination: *'What I said to myself was: "I want you to get better, you know. You've got to do something . . ."'*

If it is impossible to generate this kind of talk, either because of the aphasia, or because of overwhelming distress, it may be provided by others. By reminding him of his responsibilities, Govi's girlfriend supplied him with the 'fighting talk' he was unable to generate himself. Because she understood and acknowledged his despair, she helped him to feel less overwhelmed:

'That girl said to me: "Alright. What happened is happened. Alright? You have to adapt your life. Because what happened is happened. And you think about your . . . me . . . and about your kids." Yeah? Then I feel better, better.'

Drawing on past events

Often frustrated in their attempts at talking with and understanding others, some people may try drawing on past events to try and make sense of the experience they are going through. Edward found his bearings by thinking about when he was nearly blinded in World War II. Reflecting on this experience gave him a perspective from which to judge the experience of stroke:

'I think it's a number of things that you think . . . I mean life is a set of experiences and so therefore if you've had bad experiences you have to relate to them. I mean when in the war I was actually blinded and eventually I recovered . . . But I'm inclined to think that if you can actually see a bit and you can actually talk a bit . . . it's better than . . . so therefore the whole thing is relative — It wasn't right, but on the other hand it isn't as bad as it could have been . . .'

Sensitivity and respect from others

For some the sense of isolation, powerlessness and fear can be relieved by contact with other people, including professionals and family members, who try to understand what they are going through and acknowledge their position. This kind of positive contact can take many forms. Respect-fulness was valued by all those who experienced it. Treated with sensi-tivity, the aphasic person feels acknowledged despite sometimes being completely unable to communicate. Encounters like the one described by Lionel stand in marked contrast to the more common experience of being talked over:

'Well actually doctor, actually I'm surprised actually because the doctor actually talked to me — in hospital and talking down and I . . . something about I was trying to say um? no I don't remember exactly when but . . . er . . . um . . . the doctor answered me and I thought: "Yes, good. Yeah. Yeah."'

Comparison with others

It may be possible for people to find their bearings by watching others in the ward. Although comparing themselves with a person who seems markedly worse off makes some people feel better, it can sometimes have a depressing effect, especially if the person is very ill or distressed. For younger aphasic people, being placed in a ward full of older people can be frightening and disturbing. It can suggest that a previous way of life and identity might have disappeared. This sense of displacement is not helped if those around are members of the opposite sex:

'It was all women and it was and . . . all . . . I was the youngest person, you see, at that time there. I was forty-three years old. And it was people that was very decrepid. They were always asleep, wouldn't talk to me. No-one was interested in any football at all. No-one was interested in any sport. They didn't want to know that sort of thing.'

Fred

Sharing the experience with others in a similar situation

Meeting other people in a similar situation made Rebecca's hospital experience more bearable:

'In fact we used to cause a bit of a riot because we used to sit there and laugh our heads off at stupid things. — Well, just . . . just the situation we were all in — You know, it was just really funny . . . just the things you do and talk about when you're in hospital. There's this really peculiar situation just throws you all together and you're sort of dealing with it. You're all encouraging one other.'

The positive effect of other people's company allowed Rebecca to become more critical of what was happening to her in hospital, and to feel that she was not alone.

Problem-solving approach to communication problems

Some people have the positive experience of encountering professionals who are able to help them find a way of communicating. Even the feeling that attempts at communication are partially understood can relieve the sense of isolation imposed by aphasia:

'Someone that could . . . could . . . er . . . listen to and talk to you and understand what you're try . . . you . . . As soon as I got to the hospital and started talking to the speech therapist. She was . . . ooh . . . a wonderful person. She understood everything I was saying. I felt it was Double Dutch, but she could understand every word. I know she was trained to understand but . . . that person in herself was . . . oh . . . something that took away this big cloud over your head all the time.'

Fred

Breakthroughs like this seem to be rare and do not result from the efforts of professionals alone. Rose, who was initially only able to say the word '*No*' describes the effects of her husband's problem-solving approach:

'I had no way of communicating with the outside world and suddenly, my husband, bless his cotton socks, um . . . thought that if I answered "No" for "No" and "No no no no no" for "Yes" then that would break it. And that did that er . . . I mean half the time, three quarters of the time broke it. And then I was instantly . . . I mean just so grateful, so . . . I mean the tiny glimmer of hope just pierced the way forward . . .'

Keeping up appearances

By keeping up appearances, some aphasic people attempt to show that they are still intelligent, despite having difficulties with language. This can be done in a number of ways. Rob and Jenny found that laughing at their aphasic errors helped to show people that they were aware of what was happening, although often they weren't really amused: *'I've treated it as a joke sometimes. You laugh . . . Sometimes it hurts . . . I think I don't really think it's funny although I'm laughing.'* Jenny developed other strategies to avoid showing herself up:

'Sometimes when it comes out . . . you know it sounds silly but it's out so there's nothing you can do about that once it goes out — You feel so silly you just shut up, think: "I won't say that in case the same thing's going to happen."'

Kiran found that reading, or at least appearing to read, was a useful way of keeping in touch with his old self, and signalling his intelligence to other people, when it was impossible to do this through speaking:

'My brother-in-law . . . my wife got me The Guardian *to read, almost from day one — And I was glad to have* The Guardian *to read — I could see the words made sense, but not to me — I was glad that I got* The Guardian *delivered but I could not read it — It signified that there was no problem. Er . . . I was used to* The Guardian.*'*

Starting to cope with illness and aphasia

- Using fighting talk.
- Drawing on past experiences.
- Being treated with respect, dignity and sensitivity, especially by those concerned with medical care.
- Comparison with others.
- Sharing the experience with others in a similar situation.
- Problem-solving approach to communication difficulties.
- Keeping up appearances.

Returning home

Leaving hospital and returning home is a significant event for anyone who has been ill. It can seem to be a sign that recovery is well on the way and everything is going to be alright. As such, the experience of coming home can bring an initial sense of relief. Away from the routines of hospital life, some aphasic people may feel they are able to focus on regaining the language they have lost:

'I'm much better at home. I'm much better. I'm . . . I was much better walking the common and saying: "house' " er . . . er . . . "wall". You know it . . . you know . . . "green" or "blue" you know.'

Edward

The sense of optimism which many people experience at the point of returning home seems to arise from how they view their condition at the time. The dramatic nature of the stroke, together with the experience of being in hospital and being treated as a patient can strengthen an impression that what has happened is a short-term illness, from which they will soon recover. For those who want to look ahead, this way of seeing things can fuel positive thoughts about the future:

'I kept saying in my way er . . . er . . ."Give me six months and I'll be back to work." — I thought it was like having a cold, flu, or something like that . . .'

Alf

But the joy of returning home can often be short-lived as people are confronted with the everyday reality of their limitations, together with the reminders of what they have lost. People respond to this time in a number of different ways. Initial feelings of joy, optimism and determination soon become tempered by other feelings.

Feelings on returning home

- *'. . . exhilarated, exhilarated.'*
- *'put that behind me and start again.'*
- *'I just couldn't do anything.'*
- *'I thought this is the end.'*
- *'My wife says I was terrible to get on with at that time.'*
- *'I see my wife working. I upset really.'*
- *'It made me bawl me eyes out every time I couldn't do it.'*
- *'I was getting frightened by me . . . indoors.'*
- *'I don't know what I'm supposed to be doing today.'*
- *'I was . . . I wouldn't say helpless, but dumped.'*
- *'Give me six months and I'll be back at work.'*

Physical impairments at home

Strong feelings can surface as people encounter the restrictions of physical impairment in their homes. For many, these become immediately obvious as they face steps and stairs, narrow doorways and inaccessible toilets. Aggravated by these restrictions and often having to wait weeks and maybe months for aids and adaptations, many aphasic people who have physical impairments find their frustration becomes mixed with anxiety about the strain placed upon partners and family members who are trying to help them:

'I felt really low and I thought: "Well, this is the end" and it really worried me — . And of course, my wife was not a strong person, by any means, and tried to get me up the steps in the wheelchair —. It was horrible, being pushed about you know. And I was always frightened that something would happen to her, her straining and all that. — I was frightened how am I going to get down?'

Ted

Communication impairment at home

Being back at home also allows people who have aphasia to realise, perhaps for the first time, the full impact of the communication impairment. While in hospital, they are, to a certain extent, cushioned from the demands of everyday communication: the phone calls which have to be made, the messages to be jotted down, the cheques to be made out. At home, as they start to re-enter the routines of shopping, dealing with the household mail and talking with neighbours and acquaintances in the street, their difficulties with language become exposed:

'And, like, chatting and chatting and chatting and cha . . . And like, it's like, hope and pray, is like, walk away, walk away but is they not walk away just sit and . . . er like I just what can I . . . Is like me speech is just tongue-tied. Tongue-tied, like out on the street is just . . . what can I say . . . is just . . .'

Stephen

Being at home also means that aphasic people have to start using their own time, instead of having it filled for them by the routines of work or hospital. They are thrown on their own resources and it quickly becomes apparent how aphasia can make it difficult to plan and arrange. The sense of uncertainty about what to do with the day can be frightening:

'Is er . . . just . . . wake up and er . . . just horrible. I mean, just, like two or three months is like . . . like the curtains. Is er . . . just terrible. I want to go out, like, shopping, anything. But is quite scary.'

Stephen

'Long, hard struggle'

The early experience of stroke and aphasia exposes many people to what will become major issues in their lives. In the unfamiliar hospital environment, they have to start the business of getting over the shock of illness and gradually recovering without having the language to ask for and understand information about their condition and its treatment. For some, this time represents the start of many months' work, as they attend the various therapies which they are not always able to understand. Often because they are unable to exert any control over what is happening, they experience feelings of uncertainty, anxiety, fear, and anger. They have to deal with the major losses and anxieties incurred by the stroke on their own. Isolated and cut off, they feel vulnerable and powerless as they encounter a range of reactions from other people, from the sympathetic and respectful, to the ignorant and discriminatory. They start to develop ways of coping with their loss of language.

In many cases, these early experiences can set the pattern for the following years. All of the issues raised in this chapter will reappear throughout the course of this book as it documents the experience of learning to live with aphasia. This begins as people leave the structured routines of hospital life and return home — often a difficult as well as joyful experience. It is the point at which many feel confronted by their previous lifestyle and start to pick up the threads which have been so suddenly left down.

3

'The thing is — what job?':
work, leisure and aphasia

On returning home, the aphasic person starts to pick up some of the threads of everyday life. During this period, while rehabilitation and therapies are usually still on-going, many seek to re-establish the patterns which structured life before aphasia, in the form of domestic roles, relationships and the familiar routines of work and relaxation. But these everyday patterns and rhythms can alter dramatically following a stroke.

Figure 3.1 shows the patterns of employment, before and after stroke, of the fifty aphasic people who took part in this study. As it concerns only a small number of people, the information does not statistically represent what happens with the employment of the aphasic population as a whole. Nevertheless, it indicates the dramatic changes which can take place. The majority were in some form of paid employment at the time of their stroke. The rest were retired, unemployed, working in a voluntary capacity or doing unpaid work in raising a family, running a household or caring for invalid relatives. Following the onset of aphasia, only one person, the youngest in the study, returned to the same employment as before on a full-time basis. A few found part-time work. The rest became unemployed or retired, depending on their age and circumstances. This chapter will focus on how and why such marked changes in patterns of work take place, and how people deal with them.

'That's it. Finished.': deciding about work

Some aphasic people move smoothly towards reaching a clear and independent decision about whether or not to return to work:

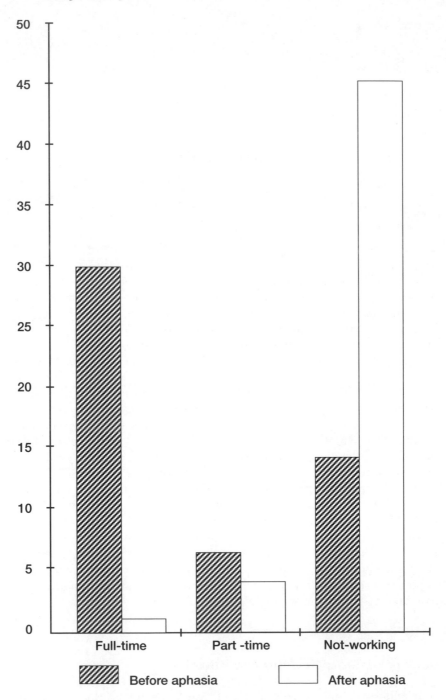

Figure 3.1. Changes in working status

'It was only about four or five months. I cannot use my right hand. I cannot talk to people on the phone. "No", I said.'

Mike

'About January I think: "No. That's it. Finished." '

Susan

Others, like Christopher, can only reach their decision when they have put themselves through the painful experience of attempting to work as before:

Working as an engineer for an aeronautical firm, **Christopher** was 33 when he had a stroke, which left him with some physical weakness and moderately severe aphasia. His job was *'relatively complicated'*, involving computer programming, mathematics and other technical skills. Three months after his stroke, Christopher was convinced that he would be able to return to work and was anxious to do this in order to continue supporting his young family. He persuaded his GP that this was possible: *'I said to the doctor: "I will get back to work." '* The doctor seemed doubtful, but didn't try to dissuade Christopher from his belief. Six months after his stroke, Christopher went to see his boss and persuaded him to let him try some programming: *'I told him my predicament and I said: "Could I borrow a spec . . . a specification?" — Because this was the specification I used to programme a computer software. And I couldn't do it. — I thought I could do it and I . . . thought I could do it and . . . then again it wasn't surprising. — That event told me I could never do it again.'* Christopher did not return to his job. He now runs the household and cares for his two sons, while his wife works full-time. He is currently thinking about the possibility of earning money from making furniture.

Christopher's account suggests the complex combination of factors which affect whether or not a person who has aphasia returns to work. These fall into two main groups. First, there are factors which are external to the aphasic person. These include the opportunities, alternatives and support which are available, and the decisions made and advice given by others, including doctors and employers. Such influences can have a powerful effect on what happens. Doctors, employers and others can take the initiative in raising the issue of the return to work and reviewing the options available. These may include the changing or reducing work, early retirement and the uptake of benefits, pensions and redundancy packages.

Other factors concern the degree to which the person understands the nature and severity of the aphasia and the other effects of stroke. In order to reach a decision, the aphasic person needs to be able to acknowledge how job performance is likely to be affected. This means becoming familiar with the limitations imposed by aphasia together with other consequences such as physical weakness and fatigue, and understanding that these are likely to be long-term problems. Those whose work was highly dependent on their communication skills, for example teachers, shop assistants and secretaries, may find that they quickly reach the understanding that returning to the same form of work is unlikely. Others, for whom communication was less important, or whose language is less impaired, may need more time to appreciate exactly what the implications are.

Proud that he never had a sick day in his 29 years as an electrician and handyman, **Vincent** found it difficult to tolerate the inactivity imposed by his stroke, especially given the fact that he had little physical impairment. Vincent became impatient with his speech and language therapy because: *'All my theory was get back to work.'* However, his doctor warned him that returning to work might be dangerous for his health. He wasn't told, and did not find out about benefits he could claim, partly because his aphasia made it difficult for him to explore his options, and partly because he felt this was wrong: *'I never intend to live off the state.'* Nevertheless, he was worried about how his large family could be supported on his wife's income alone. He felt guilty seeing his wife working when he was doing nothing. He couldn't accept the changes in his long-established working pattern. He felt that his sense of identity was under threat, and he became depressed: *'It was should me going to work.'* A year after his stroke, he allowed himself to acknowledge that things were not going to get better: *'I was dependent on myself and not the state. Those thing used to hit me for the first year. I would say eighteen months. And I keep on thinking . . . then I discovered and said: "Well, the time is pass. You not going to get it better." So . . . so if somebody had come up . . . maybe information what I would have need, which I don't know, maybe would have helped me. Maybe people know the information what they give me but they didn't make any effort.'* Being near retirement age anyway, Vincent did not return to full-time work but busied himself with running the household. He occasionally does casual work for friends.

The process of reaching a decision is complicated by the aphasic person's attitudes towards work. These are determined by a number of factors, including the point reached in working life, how much working was valued and enjoyed, the degree of financial responsibility carried, the level of awareness of alternatives and support systems, feelings about seeking financial help and personal fears and qualms, for example about how workmates might react to the changes in communication. Thus, for someone who is nearing retirement age and who can anticipate the benefits of a mature pension scheme, the motivation to return to work may not be high. For someone who is starting or settling into a career, who identifies strongly with their work or who, like Christopher, carries the burden of financial responsibility for a family, the drive to return may be overwhelming. Such influences can make it difficult to think clearly about the effects of aphasia.

Whether or not the decision not to stop work has been reached smoothly, it can be painful. Giving up, for some, means having to do without stimulation, a social network, money, prestige and interest. This can lead to some feelings of bitterness:

'Got no job at all now. That hurts. Hurts a lot, you know. — Angry really. Why me? Good job and all.'

Philip

However, attitudes to stopping work are not always straightforward. It can be a relief to give up a gruelling, difficult or tedious job. Those who are near retirement age, or who have felt the threat of redundancy may be ready to stop and have already prepared themselves somewhat for the change of pace. Feelings may be ambivalent, in that it is possible to regret the loss of some aspects of a job and yet feel glad to be free of others. Thus, stimulation, prestige, money and company may be missed, but not stress, fatigue and tedium.

Finding alternatives

If returning to the same work as before on a full-time basis becomes impossible after a stroke, the experience of those who took part in this study suggests that a number of alternatives may be possible.

Pathways to working after aphasia

- Adapting work patterns.
- Changing jobs.
- Education/training.
- Re-training.
- Voluntary work.

Adapting work patterns

It may be possible, with the support of a sympathetic employer, to resume work on a part-time basis and to modify both the timing and the nature of the work undertaken to meet the aphasic person's needs and abilities. Mark's experience is an example of how this can work.

Mark is gradually increasing the number of hours he spends at work in an office administering a hospital hairdressing service. He is adapting his role to suit his needs and abilities. He has stopped dealing with phone calls to the office because of his aphasia. However, he is taking on more standard letter writing: *'I know I am typing fairly well . . . Um . . . "Thank you for the letter of the first instance. I'm enclosing our first invoice for the next month's hire period. There is no increase in our annual inflation which remains at £121". . . blah, blah, blah.'* Mark is able to work the hours which suit him, to build up his attendance gradually, and to adapt his work to suit his language needs and abilities. He and his employer are removing obstacles to his employment by changing both the timing and the nature of his work. Mark is employed by his father.

Others are not so lucky. There is little other evidence of awareness of the barriers faced by aphasic people who wish to work. Commitment to employing disabled workers appears to be realised, if at all, in terms of improving physical access. The majority experience suggests that the nature and impact of aphasia is not recognised or understood by employers. In addition, their language impairment can place aphasic people in a double-bind, by hindering them from putting forward a case for modified employment.

In the United Kingdom, one option for returning to modified employment is to negotiate this as part of rehabilitation, limiting income to 'therapeutic earnings'. Under this scheme, a certain amount (in 1997, up to £45.50 per week) may be earned, if it is agreed that the work is likely to be therapeutically beneficial. This does not affect the person's claim on incapacity benefit or severe disablement allowance. However, arranging this seems to be no easy task as it depends, in part, on the ability of the person to put forward a persuasive and persistant case that the work is therapeutically beneficial. Even finding out who to approach for information about the guidelines regarding therapeutic earnings can be difficult. Challenging for someone with unimpaired language, such a process can prove trying for someone with aphasia:

'It's very difficult to get in touch with the people in charge with . . . of my benefits to make sure it's alright to go back as a therapy but they just sort of said: "No"

and then "You've got to write off again." And they said: "We'll think about it." And it's not very . . . I don't think the benefit . . . benefits . . . it's not very good.'

Trevor

Changing jobs

It may not be possible to adapt a job which is heavily dependent on communication skills to meet the needs and abilities of the aphasic person. An alternative to adapting the nature and timing of work is to find a different job, which is more accessible. But it can be difficult to predict exactly what the demands, and the pitfalls, will be. A new job can reveal aspects of the aphasia which were not anticipated.

Prior to his stroke, **Kiran** enjoyed the influence, prestige and demands of his post as a senior teacher. His love of working with children has led him back to work, part-time, as a general classroom assistant. He made the decision to do this after a painfully honest appraisal of his remaining language skills. It still hurts to be reminded of his previous powers and his retained abilities: *'In my present post I can see teachers making perhaps the wrong decisions for the children. I can pick it up like that. But as a classroom assistant, I have to keep my mouth shut.'* Kiran's decision to work as a classroom assistant doesn't just mean he has to restrain himself from drawing on previous experience and skills. It also means he loses money, as he is £100 a month worse off than when he was claiming benefits. His new job, while much less demanding than his previous post, is also revealing the limitations imposed by his aphasia: *'I'm perfectly capable of making decisions, but I can't have too many ideas at once. — Obviously, I cannot manage kids. I know that now. In that I tend to take slightly longer than most teachers and adults do in reacting to a given situation. By the time I react, the incident is over.'* He is wondering about the possibility of re-training to teach adults. But re-training also poses problems for someone with aphasia, as Kiran discovered when he started a course in counselling. He did well on the course but found himself struggling to write the required essays. The special needs tutor to whom he turned for help failed to understand what aphasia was, what it meant for Kiran, what his needs were and what solutions to the problems there might be. He gave inaccurate information about computer software which might have eased one aspect of the problem, and laced this with racist remarks. Kiran gave up the course.

Education and training after aphasia

Embarking on an educational, vocational or training course may be an option, but poses specific challenges to someone who has aphasia. The process of education is generally conducted through spoken and written language. Students are required, among other things, to follow lectures, take part in seminars, tutorials and debates, read set material, take notes, produce written course work and sit exams. Aphasia can restrict the person's ability to meet these requirements. Difficulties coping with the content and meeting the demands of a course can be worsened, for someone with aphasia, by a rapid pace of teaching, and by pressures and time limits on exams and essays.

An aphasic student has special needs. The fact that these are generally not understood can cause the aphasic person to become discouraged, and give up. Kiran's experience is by no means uncommon. Because aphasia is unfamiliar to many people, including teachers and special needs tutors, the aphasic person may have to explain what it is, and what adaptations are needed. However, some accounts show how it is possible for the needs of aphasic students to be understood and met:

Rose is training to be a clinical psychologist, and has several years of part-time education ahead of her before she achieves her goal of working with people with language impairment. *'It's just a narrow road that I've got to go down before I get to the end where all these other people are standing with their hands over their mouths.'* Rose is the only one of those interviewed who is undergoing vocational training. This does not seem to be because aphasic people lack ideas or ambition, but because opportunities to undergo education or training with proper and appropriate help seem limited. Written and spoken language is crucial to education. Most educational courses expect students to read books and papers, to attend lectures, to discuss and write about their topic. Clearly, this is demanding for people with aphasia. Rose finds that studying psychology part-time through the Open University allows her the extra time she needs for reading and writing. Her tutors are sympathetic and she has contact with a special counsellor employed by the University. She is allowed extra time for essays and for exams, which she takes at home, the University providing an invigilator. She uses a word-processor to write her exams, and can therefore eliminate spelling errors. Nevertheless, she finds the process stressful, and describes how the aphasia still gets between her and the precision she would like to use in expressing her ideas: *'In my exam at first I wrote it as normal and then the aphasia started to take over and then it became so disabling that I just*

> *wasn't able to write it down. And I mean I'd skirt round the edges and I wouldn't be able to write it exactly down and oh it was just so irritating. — You want to do so well and I didn't feel I was doing myself justice . . .'* Probably no special provision would enable Rose to express herself as precisely as she would like and to meet her own high standards. Nevertheless, she continues to do well in exams and course work. She progresses through the course, feeling supported by the attention which has been given to her needs.

Some accounts in this study show how teaching methods can be adapted in a number of ways to accommodate aphasic people. For example, the use of handouts and tape-recorders in class reduce the need for note-taking. Aphasic students benefit from being given extra time to complete essays and being able to do exams at their own pace in a suitable environment. A flexible approach allows course work to be drafted, edited and proof-read in stages. Successful students also learn to pace their work and not to overload themselves. However, while some aphasic people describe how they have benefited from such measures, they are not commonly experienced. One account of a government sponsored retraining scheme shows how easily things can go wrong for the student or trainee who has aphasia. In this case, because his needs were not understood or met the aphasic trainee quickly became demoralised and abandoned the scheme.

Education and training after aphasia: factors contributing to success

- Understanding of the nature of aphasia and the aphasic person's needs and abilities.
- Course information which is easily obtained and can be understood.
- Suitable and accessible venue and time for the course.
- Choice of appropriate course/training module.
- Flexible time-scale and pacing of course requirements.
- Flexible and creative teaching methods: problem solving.
- Appropriate and informed support from special needs adviser.
- Flexibility in methods of examining and evaluating performance.
- Assertiveness and clarity on the part of the aphasic person in explaining requirements.
- Encouragement to adapt working methods.

Voluntary work

Aphasia may make it impossible to return to work or to continue with previous voluntary activities. But their experience of aphasia makes some people aware of the problems of others, and keen to offer help and support. Aphasic people may be invited to act as helpers by therapists or volunteers who are running groups. Many become committed to supporting others. Their accounts show that voluntary involvement with others can cross the spectrum of formality, from regular work with groups to the occasional visit to a newly aphasic person in hospital. Sometimes they become self-appointed guides and advisers to others struggling with aphasia. It seems that, although aphasia can sweep away previous occupations, it can also provide a focus for new personal development. Helping others with aphasia, through sharing experiences and offering advice, can bring a welcome sense of mission and purpose:

'I mean it's my most important purpose in life . . . um . . . aphasia. I would go anywhere to do it. Anything I could. — Obviously if anybody asked me if I could go to somebody who'd had a stroke I'd go quickly, you know and take my little journal with me and give them hope, I hope and . . . I mean somebody said: "Oh you are a saint," and I said: "I'm not. It's just what I have to do."'

Judith

Paula is 56 and was working as a midwife before she started her family of seven children. She was doing a part-time Open University degree in Economics when she had a stroke which left her with a marked aphasia. Now her children have reached the point of leaving home, Paula feels it is important to think about work again: *'Taken time. Sit down. The house is fine and my children are . . . one child. I don't . . . I . . . I empty.'* She is thinking about trying to become a volunteer visiting people who have had strokes: *'The volunteer . . . with some . . . some hospital'* even though she knows her limited speech would make this hard. She feels that seeing the progress she has made would encourage those in the early stages of stroke: *'I could helpful for you, for myself . . . my speech and my hands helpful. — You look at me and my speech . . . my speech and my hands better and all confidence.'* Paula is also doing a word-processing course, and is considering the possibility of trying to write a book about her experience: *'Book. Little, little.'*

Paula describes a sense of emptiness in her life now that her work of raising a family is nearing completion, an experience shared by many people as they go through life-changing events such as retirement, redundancy or the departure of children. Clearly, alterations in working patterns have a major impact on the amount of spare time available. When such changes happen because of aphasia, not only the balance, but the dynamics of work and relaxation can be affected.

'I express me I me painting': aphasia and leisure-time

Aphasia affects the dynamics of leisure and relaxation in a number of ways. First, because opportunities for working can become restricted, people with aphasia may find they have an increased amount of leisure-time on their hands. In common with those who are made redundant or retire, they can no longer enjoy the structure and contrast offered by a clearly delineated working week. Many miss the pleasure of unwinding at the end of each working day, and the enjoyment of a weekend enhanced by knowledge that work will start again on Monday morning.

Aphasia can also limit participation in certain types of leisure activity which are dependent on the use of language. It can also prompt the adaptation of old interests, and the development of new, more accessible ones. Although aphasia can affect relaxation time in these ways, its impact is by no means clear-cut and predictable. This largely depends on the type of activities undertaken in spare time prior to the stroke, and their relative importance for each person.

Use of leisure time before aphasia

The aphasic people who took part in this study occupied their pre-stroke spare time with many types of interests ranging from the sporting to the sedentary, from the sociable to the solitary. Many simply counted being with friends and family as their main way of relaxing, either at home, meeting up to go shopping, or at pubs and clubs. Woodwork, reading, watching television, knitting, do-it-yourself, gardening and cooking numbered among home interests. Sporting interests included golf, sailing, walking, fishing, bowling and football. More cultural activities included reading, writing, theatre-going, photography, dancing and music. Several people were involved in voluntary activities, for example, teaching literacy, leading a scout-troop and coaching a football team. Some were engaged in studying subjects of interest at evening classes or on a part-time basis. Most spare-time activities involved a major social component. Attending functions at the Masonic Lodge, taking part in a writing group, going to a football match and playing bowls, bingo and dominoes all offered opportunities to mix with others and to meet friends.

Attitudes to leisure time varied almost as much as the interests themselves. Some people focused on specific interests, which they pursued with concentrated attention. In some cases, these assumed such central importance that they started to take on the characteristics of work in terms of the time and attention they demanded. Other people took a more casual approach, enjoying a wide range of informal interests. For a small minority, a pressurised work schedule meant there was little time for relaxing and developing other interests:

'Five years ago as busy as ever, very busy morning, night, er . . . morning, morning, afternoon and evening. Out every time you know.'

Lionel

'It's a bit scare': factors affecting the use of spare time in aphasia

Once the processes of illness and and the rituals of rehabilitation recede, lives which have previously been filled with work can seem open and unstructured. Some aphasic people try to enquire about, arrange and participate in new activities but these can highlight the loss of language. Spending time with friends and family makes demands upon language. It is even necessary for seemingly passive and solitary occupations, such as watching television. In compromising language, aphasia can become one of the major obstacles to a full and constructive use of spare time. Of course, it does not operate alone, but in combination with a number of other factors.

Obstacles to the use of spare time in aphasia

- Language impairment.
- Physical factors.
- Financial factors.
- Attitudinal factors.
- Organisational factors.

Aphasia as an obstacle

Some ways of relaxing and spending spare time seem to be particularly vulnerable to aphasia in that they are dependent upon language. Chatting to friends, writing letters, reading magazines and books are all activities which depend upon language, and which may have to be modified or forgone:

'I always used to read a book in the evening — before I went to bed sort of thing but I haven't since I had the stroke. And it gets after about a page or so it gets so I

just . . . I just don't understand what I'm reading sort of thing. And reading about a page a night, and one book's . . . well . . . too much. I just can't. I tried . . . I just couldn't . . . can't do it.'

Trevor

As well as being enjoyed in their own right, reading, listening, writing and talking are also tools which are commonly used in the process of learning, either independently or in a class. The strain placed upon their language causes many aphasic people to abandon classes or to be fearful about taking them up. For example, Sharon would like to study astrology:

'Me . . . thinking about which one of er . . . the evening . . . class, but . . . um . . . I like the stars and things — planets and stuff but um reading and writing is bad and um . . . all the time I'm thinking ordinary people visits the class and writing and thinking about the things er . . . do . . . well the language or stuff. But oh God it's too much.'

Because aphasia can specifically weaken the ability to find the name of items, interests which involve identification and labelling can be particularly vulnerable. This can be aggravating, especially if the main focus of the activity falls on selecting the correct name from all the options. Roger describes how aphasia affects two of his previous interests: bird watching and collecting plants. He can recognise what he sees, but cannot find the correct names:

'What's the name of so and so? — My son take me on the lake there. The birds there. The birds there . . . recognise the birds. Name things . . . not even the birds. No I can't. — The trouble me, see, forget the words. Like all the um . . . like er . . . garden, flowers.'

Aphasia does not affect specific leisure pursuits in isolation. It can also impair the ability to fulfil roles and take part in the social interactions connected with or central to an interest. Thus, the captain of a domino team, who is still able to play, becomes reluctant to continue in that role because this involves making speeches and he feels he no longer knows what to say. The woman who used to give regular dinner parties now doubts her ability to entertain guests with anecdotes and funny stories. The woman who used to enjoy meeting her friends in the pub can no longer deal with a noisy environment and conversation which moves too quickly between too many people. The regular church-goer and fundraiser finds the post-service chatter difficult to join with and starts to cut himself off.

Thus, aphasia can affect many different aspects of leisure and relaxation and can force people to change how they take part, or to withdraw from an activity or interest.

Physical obstacles

Many aphasic people experience the loss of leisure interests and pursuits because of physical impairment. This can be the case even for those with no paralysis, but who experience other physical effects following the stroke, for example chronic fatigue or impaired co-ordination.

Paralysis, weakness, fatigue and loss of mobility and co-ordination will inevitably affect participation in some forms of active sport such as golf and football, and pursuits such as ballroom dancing. Poor access to public transport, to museums, football grounds, galleries, cinemas, pubs, cafes, restaurants and theatres can become a major barrier for those who have a significant physical impairment. Post-stroke epilepsy, poor co-ordination and weakness can make it unsafe for the aphasic person to drive, limiting many activities. Such losses can be hard to bear, especially for those whose identity is determined as much by their interests and activities as by their work and relationships.

Financial barriers

Limited opportunities for work and dependence on benefits means that many aphasic people experience a drop in income. This can have a knock-on effect on the maintenance of costly leisure pursuits. Living within new and restricted means, it may become impossible to afford items such as golf club membership fees, a personal computer, a taxi fare, a tankful of petrol, a round of drinks at a pub, course fees, a fishing licence, garden plants and photographic equipment. Often, cost factors combine with other factors to limit social and leisure activities.

Betty's active social and leisure life has changed dramatically since her stroke, for a number of reasons. Aphasia means she can no longer write stories and articles as before, and also makes it difficult for her to participate in the discussions at her writers' group: *'I'm going to the writing club tomorrow all being well, and naturally they talk backwards and forwards . . . er . . . erudite discussions and if I want to speak I lift my hand up . . . very good about that and I er . . . speak. But by the time I've got it, you know, the thought has gone.'* She finds that her aphasia limits her to reading popular fiction: *'I've got this place is full of books. — Um, the Agatha Christie I used to read yards of them when I was ill or sleep and now I read them over and over again.'* Unable to continue supplementing her income through writing articles, and living on a small pension from her work and her savings, Betty faces many restrictions. She knows her writing would be easier if she could use a word-processor instead of her old typewriter. But this is beyond her reach financially: *'I make so much mistakes and the computer can erase them without having to go through thing again. — I should have had it years ago if I could have afforded it.'* Betty finds herself withdrawing from social contact partly because of her aphasia and partly because of the money involved: *'My social life has gone down because a) I don't want to and b) I can't afford it. I can't even afford a paper in the morning.'* Not being able to afford a paper further reduces her confidence in her abilities to converse knowledgeably with her friends. She also had to give up her car because she couldn't afford to maintain it and because she became alarmed by the traffic. This also restricts her social life as she is dependent on public transport, which can be expensive, or on friends offering her a lift. Betty is supported by her friends in attending the writers' group and participating in the discussions. Despite the fact that she is taking part, she finds the experience depressing because it points up how much she has changed. She feels she is no longer the witty, erudite, verbal person she used to be.

Attitudinal barriers

Betty expresses distress at the erosion of the aspects of her identity which were concerned with writing and talking. This is a feeling shared by many aphasic people. Embarrassment, a sense of incompetence, depression and loss of confidence can act as barriers to the uptake of leisure pursuits just as much as the technical loss of language imposed by aphasia. Like Betty, many people feel that the restrictions on their reading, language and their lifestyle mean that they may have little of value to contribute to meetings and conversations with others.

Feelings of anxiety about possible incompetence mingle with fear about other people's reactions to the aphasia. This can make it difficult to pick up favourite pursuits like going to the pub, especially when the stress of putting in an order at the bar can instantly make the aphasia seem worse:

'Even today now I lunch once a week with the wife. Go to the bar and nothing comes out. People are looking and they say: "What's wrong with this man?" But it soon wears off after a while. You can get . . . oh I can get by anywhere now but as I say, people do think you're drunk.'

Fred

Organisational barriers

Aphasic people can encounter a number of organisational barriers in seeking to maintain or develop their leisure interests. Some of these can be practical, for example finding an activity which is located near to home and which takes place at a suitable time of day. The other type of organisational barrier concerns getting information, a process which can be particularly weakened by aphasia. Knowing they have to find out about an appropriate course, club or class, check the venue, cost, time and negotiate a place can discourage a person who has aphasia, even from making some preliminary enquiries. Organisational problems also combine with aphasia to affect other types of activities. For example, arranging to meet with friends may involve a number of language-based processes including ringing round, checking dates, noting times, locating venues and registering changes in arrangements.

At any number of points in this process, things can go wrong. In terms of setting up attendance on a course, it may be difficult to give information about the needs resulting from the aphasia and to understand information about what is offered. One aphasic person who took part in this study wanted help with his spelling and found himself about to be registered on a course for people with learning disabilities. Those whose language is unimpaired find such organisational problems aggravating. For the person with aphasia, who perhaps has to plan and rehearse every phone call, they can present a daunting prospect.

This is perhaps the reason why few aphasic people seem to take an active part in re-organising their leisure time. Many are glad to take the chance to develop interests and relationships which become available to them through therapies, day centres and stroke clubs, precisely because they are pre-organised, available and accessible. These opportunities can offer new experiences and the chance to develop new interests and skills.

'Got more enjoyment': passing time with aphasia

Many people with aphasia are able to find ways of using the extra time released if they stop work or have to give up previous interests.

Adapting leisure interests

Several examples are given of ways in which interests can be maintained in a modified form despite the presence of physical impairment. These examples form a useful parallel to adaptations which meet the language abilities of an aphasic person. Thus the sports fanatic while *'sad, very sad'* that he is unable to play football as before, finds that, despite his right-sided weakness, he is able to play table tennis and pool, albeit with a modified style. The ex-county bowler now plays skittles at her local stroke club. These changes can allow a certain amount of reconnection with aspects of the former self as Govi, a passionate driver, indicates:

'I got a car adapted for me. And er . . . car is very necessary. I used to drive when I was six year old. — My girlfriend got everything for me. You have to give test. — It's not a very easy. No. — After five months in hospital I told her: "I can drive". But er . . . then I take my time because I know it's . . . I was . . . I want to er . . . I was . . . how to put it? . . . dying to drive. Yeah, yeah. Because my whole life was in driving also. Er . . . it's because I can't live without car.'

In a similar way, interests can sometimes be adapted to accommodate the change in language abilities. Those who used to enjoy reading sometimes find that this interest can be maintained using tape-recorded books. Difficulty following complex knitting patterns does not mean that an interest in handicrafts has to be abandoned. Tapestry work, for example, involves the ability to match shapes and colours without language, yet the end result can be just as intricate, skillful and satisfying. Previously intense social contact can be wound down in the more flexible and relaxed atmosphere of the club-house bar:

'I can actually engage in conversations and then, you know, I can withdraw or whatever.'

Edward

Some people find that they can adapt their interest and delight in literature even though it is not possible to read or listen to it with understanding. For example, Ken has a book in which he has copied out the poetry he used to love reading. For him, it was worth the effort of doing this to reconnect himself with what he cannot now fully understand. Similarly, learning copy-typing or the principles of word-processing can make written language feel more accessible.

Development of new interests

Marked language difficulties can limit or change participation in leisure activities which are heavily dependent on language. Many aphasic people in these circumstances find themselves learning new skills which by-pass the need for language more or less altogether. Painting, pottery, woodwork, engraving, listening to music and flower-arranging are all activities which have been taken up by those with marked language impairments. Many of these activities can be demonstrated and taken up virtually without language and are often part of the repertoire of activities available at day centres. For someone like Jack, who has severe aphasia, painting has become a lifeline. He says:

'I express me I me painting.'

A small number of people with aphasia may find that they develop new interests as a result of their experience of aphasia and its treatment. It is possible to become fascinated with the subject of language impairment, and choose to study it in more depth. Some wish to place their own experience on record, perhaps through writing. An interest in supporting other aphasic people can expand into voluntary work and bring opportunities to develop new friendships and new forms of social life. Exposure, perhaps for the first time, to the use of word-processors and computers which are increasingly used in therapy, may open up new vistas of interest for someone with aphasia:

'Like . . . like eight years ago it's: "Computing? Got to be joking. No chance."
And now, like now, like four, five years ago, it's a: "Well I suppose so." Is learn
the keyboard and like I quite enjoy it. Quite enjoy it.'

Stephen

'I haven't any life': reactions to changes in lifestyle

Aphasic people experience a wide variety of reactions to changes in their patterns of work and relaxation. Some people are overwhelmed by their losses and find it difficult to move on from a sense of bitterness, grief and regret. At the other extreme there are those who feel that their appreciation and enjoyment of life has been enhanced, either by the experience of surviving a stroke, or by the freedom which has opened up for them as a result of it. They intensely appreciate ordinary, everyday pursuits.

'I'm very satisfied with what I do.'

Douglas

'I think to myself: "Oh thank God I can watch the telly."'

Pearl

The middle ground is taken up by those who acknowledge their losses and are saddened by them, but who tolerate and make the best of their situation:

Madge used to be fully occupied with working, caring for her elderly mother and conducting an active social life prior to her stroke: *'I had such a life before. I had a man friend and I had Mum and my girlfriends. I used to go away for weekends. — I had a far busier life then.'* Following Madge's stroke, which left her unable to walk and with unclear speech and mild aphasia, her mother moved into a nursing home, where she died. Madge doesn't go out much now, except to a stroke club, and to visit her family for holidays. She could arrange to go back to her old club, but now finds it difficult to meet people who remember her as she was: *'I'm afraid I'm going to be seen by friends. Not necessarily friends, but neighbours. — I still get terrified joining in with people I know. — There are times when I've thought: "Oh I'd love to be going down the club tonight." But then it passes.'* Madge allows herself a couple of tots of whisky at night and watches television. Close friends also come and call. She finds it ironic that although she is now better off than before thanks to the Independent Living Fund, she is unable to enjoy her prosperity in the way she would like: *'Although I don't do much I don't get depressed or bored. — I do still like to drink. And I am ever so happy. — I had a far busier life then. But I wish I had certain things then . . . if I had the money I got now. I'm better off than I've ever been. But I'm not better off because I haven't got any life.'*

People who have aphasia are not the only ones who are affected by changing patterns of work and leisure. Family members, friends, employers and workmates also find themselves taking on new roles and trying to adjust to the changes brought by the stroke. The next chapter explores what happens between aphasic people and those around them when language is damaged or lost.

4

'Can I get a word in edgeways?': family, friends and aphasia

Aphasia does not just affect those who have it. The impact of language impairment is felt across entire social networks, by partners, children, parents, siblings, friends and colleagues. As aphasia settles into their lives, they are faced with changes in their relationships with the aphasic person that can be deep and long-lasting. One reason for this is that language is the currency of relationships. It is used to invite, to suggest, to question, to advise, to argue, to reprimand, to bargain, to joke and to reassure. The changing needs and attitudes of each person are expressed and responded to, largely through the medium of language. As an obstacle to the sending and receiving of such messages, aphasia reduces the influence of one person in what was once a two-way process.

This chapter will explore how losing language affects different kinds of relationships. It will trace how aphasic people, their friends and families cope with the changes in communication. However, this will all be done from the perspective of aphasic people themselves, not those around them. The experiences, comments and interpretations which make up this chapter, therefore, give only one side of the story.

'Can't comfort Helen': how aphasia affects marriage and partnership

While some partnerships and marriages have not survived, most of the aphasic people who took part in this study remain with their partners. Whether the outcome involves separation or not, a number of changes can cause stress to a partnership following stroke. These can combine to affect both partners, bringing disharmony and stress even to relationships which keep going.

> **What factors contribute to stress in partnerships following stroke?**
>
> • Changes in communication.
> • Physical changes.
> • Emotional changes.
> • Role changes.

Changes in communication

It can be very distressing for a couple to be unable to communicate, especially at a time of trauma. When one partner suddenly becomes ill with stroke, questions need to be asked, plans and arrangements need to be discussed, and reassurances given. Severe aphasia can mean that it is impossible to express basic needs, let alone fears and concerns. Those with less marked aphasia may not be able to share worries, ask questions or console an anxious partner. Stresses such as this can bring about feelings of anger, frustration, and depression. A familiar source of comfort may have dried up because reassuring words cannot be spoken or understood. It may feel as if the experience is not being shared because it can't be talked about.

Partners often develop their own strategies when trying to help the aphasic person to communicate. Those that can be helpful include addressing the aphasic person directly, and giving time to the conversation. Less helpful strategies include not allowing any attempts at speech, finishing off what the aphasic person is trying to say, speaking for or over the person, and insisting on words and phrases being repeated correctly. Although they are well intentioned, such strategies can cause frustration and rage in the aphasic person, who nevertheless may be unable to object.

Changes in communication do not just mean that the exchange of information and ideas becomes difficult. They can have effects on other aspects of the relationship, for example it may not be possible for the aphasic person to keep anything secret from the partner. Flagging communication can also impact on a couple's sexual relationship:

Interviewer: Has it affected the relationship between you and your wife . . . the speaking problem? —
Ken: Yes, yes, yes.
Interviewer: In what way?
Ken: Two beds.

Physical changes

Sexuality between partners can also be affected by physical changes which can result from stroke. Changes of appearance, body image and shape, loss of movement and sensation, fatigue and fear of exertion combine to stifle interest on both sides. Fatigue can affect both partners, especially if the person with aphasia needs a lot of physical help and support.

Rose describes some of the stresses her marriage underwent in the early days following her stroke. Virtually unable to speak, and with a weak right side, Rose's days on her return from hospital were spent caring for her new baby and her young son, with support and help from her mother-in-law and her husband. Her husband started to feel delayed effects of the shock and trauma they had both undergone. When he returned to work she found the physical changes she had undergone and her exhaustion, combined with changed patterns of communication, contributed to increasing levels of tension between them. They started to drift apart: *'He would go to work at eight and he'd come home at seven or eight and I was up with the children and go to bed with the children and so our relationship suffered of course. — I put on so much weight taking these pills and I felt hideous about myself. I mean underneath I'd be so unhappy and I kept a sort of jolly face on for all concerned. But I'd just underneath I'd feel so hideous. — He's very eloquent and very articulate and I mean, no way could I top that because he was just so overpowering. Normally, we'd hold our own but he was so overpowering he'd sort of make me feel so inadequate and so shitty. I'd feel like a live-in nanny. And that was what I felt like for two years after.'* The relationship survived this period, and the couple are now extremely close.

Emotional changes

Rose's account illustrates how physical changes and exhaustion, together with her communication losses made her feel miserable, although she struggled to conceal this. Emotional responses to a stroke can range from anger and frustration to depression. These emotions, and the swings between them, can radically affect the will to attempt communication. They are difficult for partners to handle, especially when they, too, are struggling with their own emotions, which can include anger, anxiety, guilt and grief for aspects of the person which have been lost, as Sharon suggests:

'Too much of with me disabled. — John's sense with me um angry or maybe child. — All the time yes but the made him moods. Yeah moods . . . um mood

swings oh God . . . I er . . . lethargic and crying and stuff. It was too much and all the time me normal, laugh and joke and out and about and playing and exercise . . .'

Role changes

Role changes in a partnership occur as a result of the changes in language and the other effects of a stroke. Loss of work for the aphasic person can be financially and emotionally stressful. The partner may need to find a job or move into full-time work. Some partners, both men and women, give up their own work or free time and become full-time care-givers. The days become filled with washing, feeding and lifting and all the other tasks required by someone with marked physical problems. Some take over new roles in the household, such as cooking and sorting out finances, because the aphasic person is unable to continue them. Both partners may become consumed with anxiety about their finances, and have to cope with restrictions in their lifestyle as a result of their newly limited means. The fabric of everyday life changes and both the aphasic person and the partner have to adjust to these shifts perhaps without being able to discuss them. For some, the new roles are never anything other than stressful. Others find they eventually come to accept the changed situation.

Les and his wife had a happy relationship before his stroke. They had spent much of their working life apart, as he did night shifts and she worked during the day, as well as caring for her elderly mother who had Alzheimer's disease. Their son also lived at home. After his stroke, Les was glad to stop work and was at home most of the time. His wife, strained by her existing responsibilities, had to take on the household finances, which had always been his domain. Together all the time, the couple found that tension was starting to tell: *'You got to realise it was strained. — You see, each person needs their own space. And you think to yourself: "Well a three-bedroomed house is big enough." But it isn't.'* She asked their son to leave home, a move which Les did not want at the time, but he now thinks was the right thing. After her mother died, Les's wife settled into a care-giving role and he started to feel more relaxed about the protection and help she wanted to offer him: *'She's very with it. She's been enquiring about this and that and she been able to help other people where we never had help — My wife has been the carer all the way through. — I don't take no responsibility whatsoever now. In fact when I go out I don't even carry money. Because the wife does everything.'*

'I couldn't do nothing about it': patterns of partnership in aphasia

As the aphasia becomes established and all the implications of the stroke start to unfold, both partners have to develop ways of communicating so that they can continue to deal with life events as a couple. For some, the process of relating to each other continues to be complex and ever-changing. Others settle into more predictable patterns, as levels of physical and communicative ability become clearer. Some aphasic people describe themselves being treated in a particular way by their partner in every exchange. The types of approach to the relationship taken by the non-aphasic partner are perceived to be positive and supportive at one extreme, hostile and destructive at the other.

A few people seem able to facilitate their aphasic partners, maintaining a delicate balance between the support and respect they are able to offer. While this balance is often difficult to achieve, some partners are able to convey to the aphasic person the general impression that they are loved and valued. In some cases, supportiveness changes into protectiveness, as the partner tries to shield the aphasic person from the stresses and demands of the outside world. But the loss of the ability to communicate can also lead some people to dominate their aphasic partners, taking control over every interaction and making every decision. And for a small number, aphasia can bring out negative responses. Some aphasic people find that they are consistently ignored or rejected by their partners, others that their attempts at communication are met with hostility and anger.

These patterns of relating may or may not have existed in some form in the partnership for many years before the arrival of aphasia and therefore may be familiar to the couple. Although some seem destructive and negative, this is not always the case. The patterns should not be simplistically judged, for they are ways of coping that partners work out for themselves, which enable the relationship to function. It is possible, for example, for an aphasic person to feel comfortable with being protected or very appreciative of a partner who takes over entirely. Even the response of a partner who constantly reacts to communication attempts with exasperation, fury or disdain, can become reassuringly predictable, if not exactly pleasant.

The couple who are living with aphasia face the difficult task of trying to make sure one partner's need for support in communication is met, without loss of respect and acknowledgement. What aphasia seems to do is restrict the repertoire of patterns available to the couple, so that it becomes difficult to find ways of negotiating. This is partly because negotiation requires both partners to use different, perhaps more tentative and uncertain language. But because it can remove the power to object, complain and confront as well as to negotiate, aphasia can also expose some people to exploitation.

For *Alice*, whose language is very impaired, losing money to her husband was the last straw and caused her to pull out of a troubled marriage. Her husband sorted out her benefit claim on her behalf, then spent all the money on drink, giving her one pound a week for her dinner money at the day centre she attended. More or less unable to express herself, and therefore unable to object, she decided to leave home, saving the change from her dinner money until she had enough to pay for a taxi to her daughter's house:

Alice: *Ah no. Beer. Beer. Ah yes.*
Interviewer: *He drank a lot?*
Alice: *Ah yes, yes, yes. Ah yes.*
Interviewer: *And he went quite soon after?*
Alice: *No me. — Taxi me. Yes.*

While such accounts give dramatic evidence of how things can go wrong in a partnership which is affected by aphasia, they do not convey the subtlety and complexity of the aphasic person's feelings towards a partner who is struggling with all the changes brought by stroke. Feelings can layer on top of one another, so that the same person can feel at once concerned and guilty because his partner is obviously at the end of her tether, resentful because she can't do the things which he thinks need to be done, and wary of her angry and explosive responses to him. Such complex feelings are difficult to express in a detailed way, but aspects can be simply and powerfully conveyed with very limited language: '*Mary — touchpaper.*'

Following his stroke, **Stephen** had to give up his career. His wife now works full time. She runs the household and has taken over the domestic finances, because Stephen's marked aphasia makes it difficult for him to continue with this. Although he has lost confidence in previous friendships, Stephen is able to rely on his wife as someone he can talk to. Stephen appreciates the constant support she offers him and all the work she puts into keeping the family and the relationship going: '*My wife is like a godsend.*' But, while he expresses his gratitude towards her, Stephen struggles with other, more complex emotions as he tries to describe how their relationship has changed: '*I wish the role was reversed . . . because then . . . don't get me wrong for goodness sake, is I wish anybody a stroke, but just roles reverse.*

> *Always you, Audrey, my wife and me is walking, talking and joking, but just roles reverse, a stroke. And I wonder like Audrey is . . . roles reverse is . . . I very much doubt it is the . . . um . . . How can I explain it? No, no, don't get me wrong, I love her to bits. I love her to bits — And like short temper. Is very very short. OK don't get me wrong is like Monday to Friday nine till five is tired. Very tired. Like half past five can turn the key and er: "I'm knackering absolutely — Got to have a bath." And like seven o'clock is nodding off. Is the same old tune. — All relationship is missing. Round the corner. I don't know. Maybe maybe maybe is me.'*

'The question is I can't talk': family and partnership stresses

Although many couples find ways of continuing everyday life together, times of family crisis can push the limits of the aphasic person's language. Examples of such crises include the discovery that a child is taking drugs, financial worries, serious illness of a family member, divorce and bereavement. Events like these need to be dealt with, in part, through language and communication. They highlight the fact that aphasia is not a one-off event which has limited impact, but that its effects are on-going and continuously manifesting themselves, even years after the onset. Thus, the aphasic parent who discovers his teenage daughter is addicted to heroin may be unable to understand or question the GP and discuss the situation with the family in any detail. The aphasic person whose partner becomes blind, or develops cancer or Alzheimer's disease, may have difficulty discussing the outlook or treatment. The aphasic person whose partner is dying may struggle to reassure, apologise, sort out financial matters or say goodbye.

Aphasic people who lose a partner through death or divorce are thrown on their own resources. Those used to the support or protection of a partner can find it traumatic to be confronted with managing the household, maintaining contact with family and friends and trying to re-establish an independent life.

A few weeks after she developed aphasia, **Gladys's** husband died of cancer. This relationship was the mainstay of her life. Her husband was protective towards her throughout their marriage and she still misses him. She was unable to talk fully with her husband before his death, and unable to express her grief and receive comfort afterwards. Because she had no physical impairment, and was able to continue running the household, Gladys appeared to need little help or support. She became very depressed. Five years later, her language was sufficiently improved to allow her to write down everything she wanted to say to him in a letter. She tore this up and threw it in the river as a way of saying goodbye to him. Gladys is lonely and anxious. She finds it difficult to keep established relationships going and to make new friends because of her fears about reactions to her language: *'I couldn't talk you see. That's it, yes. And I'm very, very upset about it because lots . . . I've told you some people are cruel what they say. I've been there, a lady there and I've heard her put my head away and saying: "I can't talk to her. She can't talk properly." '*

'I just sit in one side': aphasia and family relationships

Relationships with parents, brothers and sisters, cousins, and others in the family shift when someone develops aphasia. Family members can rally round, offering support and social contact to the aphasic person who may not be able to keep in touch with friends and workmates. In some cases, aphasia brings brothers and sisters, parents and children closer together and family members take the place of friends. It can even end feuds and estrangements which have gone on for years.

However, not all family members react to aphasia in a helpful way. The familiar patterns of support and protectiveness can establish themselves, as can more controlling and negative reactions. The behaviour of family members may be largely beyond the aphasic person's control. Impaired language may make it impossible for the aphasic person to ask a sister about how she is using the income from benefits. A concerned parent may unwittingly overwhelm and constrict an aphasic son or daughter, pushing an independent social life even more out of reach. A previously friendly cousin may behave in a way which seems cool and remote. The strategies developed by family members to deal with the aphasic person's communication can be as aggravating or as helpful as those developed by partners. Those who took part in this study describe many negative experiences including being unable to get a word in edgeways, and being talked over.

Relationships between aphasic people and members of their families are of course influenced by what went on between them before, and by the nature of the family culture. The person with a large, extended family, whose members all live nearby and who have always socialised together, will thus be in a very different position to the widow who has not maintained contact with her family through all the years of her marriage.

However, although it can be yearned for by someone who is isolated, plentiful company may also overwhelm the aphasic person. Because it damages language, aphasia makes it difficult to choose and control the degree and nature of contact with others.

'My family and my people, you know, like my wife's family and relatives of my wife's, and my own, you know, my . . . my friends, and my other friends, you know, they always used to come here . . . sometimes when it was so much that I had to leave them there and I go upstairs. — I my . . . family . . . they'll lose you essence, so I try very hard to forget it you know, what to say. Or I just sit in one side. Just try to ignoring.'

Ravi

'They quite often want to say: "Why?"': aphasia and relationships with children

As they progress from babyhood to adulthood, children pass through many stages each of which places different sets of demands on parents. Parents learn to cope with the ups and downs of living with the fractious toddler, the curious five-year-old, the argumentative nine-year-old and the sulky adolescent. They change their language according to the demands of the situation and yet, despite this adaptability, they are often unaware of the skill and range of the communication they use. Selecting the right language for each job, they move smoothly from episode to episode, in turn stimulating, nagging, consoling, teasing, reasoning with, calming and reprimanding their children.

Many aphasic people who took part in this study describe how feelings of love and responsibility for their children and grandchildren helped them to weather the effects of the stroke. In describing their experiences as parents and as grandparents, aphasic people are able to reveal the intricacy and subtlety of communication with children. They can talk about it precisely because they feel its loss. The following examples, drawn from accounts of relationships with children at different stages, illustrate the varying needs of offspring and some of the frustrations of aphasic parents.

The delicate process of forming a bond with a new baby is partly conducted through talking and singing to the child. This can be disrupted by a number of events, including illness and aphasia. Aphasia also makes it difficult to surface problems and ask for help, as Rose indicates when she describes coming round after her brain haemorrhage to find her baby had been delivered by Caesarean section and that she was not reacting the way people seemed to expect.

'It was a shock to me that she was my little girl. — I wanted for all the family's sake to find this instant love for her. — I think there's a definite bonding between mother and baby . . . that I just don't think I had that. It was taken away from me, purely by need, but that was taken away from me. And I remember thinking: "Well everyone's telling me I've got to cope with this baby." — But I wasn't strong enough at the time to say: "Hang on a minute. I don't want to do this and I'm not ready to do this." That was because of my language and I think if I'd had my language I'd have said exactly what I felt.'

At a later stage, some aphasic parents find they can provide the language needed by young children, and that tasks such as reading the bedtime story can help their own language to progress. But as the child matures, the demands on the parent's language become more sophisticated. Fights and arguments take place, rules are disobeyed and difficult questions are asked.

> ***Christopher's*** two sons were born after he became aphasic: *'They have never seen me as I was . . .'*. When they were little, Christopher was able to read to them, but began to find this hard as they got older and the reading matter got more difficult. Now they are aged 10 and 12 years, he feels that his aphasia means he fails to meet some of their needs. He has difficulty answering questions, explaining what words mean, helping with homework and keeping discipline. Christopher's speech is very slow, and he finds this delays his response to the younger son who *'wants to know everything immediately. — He wants me to explain everything. Why the garden grows and why the plants grow and why the . . . electricity isn't working and everything. Because that's what I'm for. I'm certain I know why but I can't get it over to them'* With the older son, Christopher feels the lack of interesting topics for discussion, partly because he is at home all day, and partly because of his aphasia: *'I got nothing to discuss with him. I would like to discuss more with him, and . . . well . . . the general family.'*

Language impairment can make it hard to help a child who is worried or in difficulties, for example, because of bullying. This is deeply distressing for the aphasic parent who desires to comfort the child and discuss the problem, but cannot find the language to do this.

A number of aphasic people who took part in the study describe experiencing conflicts with their adolescent children. They feel hurt by their moodiness and withdrawal and wonder what might be the cause. It is difficult to determine whether such behaviour is affected by the aphasia, or whether it would have happened anyway. Sometimes the withdrawal of the adolescent child from the aphasic parent does seem to be linked to the child's sense of embarrassment because the parent is 'different' or 'unusual'. Some older children of aphasic adults appear to become depressed. Aphasia does not help the parent to negotiate with the child:

'Both turned me. Both. Not easy. Not easy.'

Ken

'I couldn't communicate with him. He couldn't associate my problems with himself.'

Geoffrey

'They would look for ah . . . pushing me . . . pushing me out — because I have my speech lost.'

Paula

Parents may feel the desire to continue supporting their children, as they mature into adulthood, embark on further educational courses, select a career and perhaps find a partner. Some aphasic parents describe their regret at not being able to give their children advice as they go through these transitions. The loss of language can be particularly upsetting when traditional and ceremonial events take place.

Fred's two children were on the brink of leaving school and going to college when he became aphasic. He felt that he let them down when they needed him: *'My son was living at home but he was . . . He went off to college, you see, in between, and he needed my help a lot. My advice. I couldn't give him no help at all. That was . . . that was at the back of my mind all the time. And my daughter was . . . was . . . she was sixteen when it happened. She was on the verge of leaving school, but she went on to college as well and I couldn't help her at all on that. She had to do everything herself.'* For Fred, one of the worst consequences of his aphasia was the fact that he couldn't make a speech at his daughter's wedding: *'I can't speak profoundly. I can talk for so long and then it dries up. It's things like my daughter's wedding. I couldn't speak. I had to write it all down and my brother-in-law done it all. Talked for me. Done it all for me.'* Fred now enjoys the support and advice of his children. His son, in particular, helps him with any difficult household correspondence: *'I got him to back up.'*

Aphasic parents of adult children who live at a distance, whether in the same country or abroad, are faced with the difficulty of trying to maintain contact when writing letters and talking on the phone becomes difficult. Long-distance phone calls become expensive when speech is slow and hesitant, and the stress of the moment can make the impairment seem worse. For Amy, aphasia means she is losing touch with her daughter:

'I want to write a letter to Australia but I can't write so I can't.'

Children as care-givers

Fred's experience is one of many examples of adult offspring taking on a supportive and care-giving role to their aphasic parent. Some take on the role of care-giver full-time, providing practical and physical help. They also give help with tasks involving communication, for example finding out about benefits, dealing with tax matters, filling in forms and talking with medical staff. Most of those who receive it welcome this support, although they are wary of adding to the pressure of their offspring's busy lives. For some, though, the assistance offered by their children can feel bitter-sweet. Their children's competence drives home their own limitations, and reinforces feelings of neediness and dependence that might feel much too premature for comfort. Watching and listening to physically and linguistically able sons and daughters and hearing about achievements and ambitions, it is possible to feel jealous of all they are able to do.

Mostly, it is older children who offer support to their aphasic parents in this way, but younger children take on caring roles, too. In one extraordinary example, a two-year-old boy learnt to help his mother when she was having fits. He would put a cushion under her head, cover her with a blanket, press the helpline on the phone to contact his father, and sit holding her hand. Children who are developing language and learning to read and write often work in tandem at this with their aphasic parent. This can be difficult to accept for someone who feels responsibility for teaching their child. It can be easier for aphasic grandparents, many of whom describe the beneficial effect of being with young children. Relieved of the direct responsibility for the child's discipline and development, some grandparents seem happy to see their grandchildren as friends and peers. The accepting nature of young children can reduce their anxiety about speaking. Older children can also have a relaxing effect:

'They look after me — Same as they tell me if I've done it wrong. They laugh then. Don't tell me off or anything like that.'

Rob

'Angry about mum': aphasic people and their parents

People who have one or both parents living at the time they develop aphasia are faced with the same dilemmas regarding this relationship as those whose language is intact. Attitudes to parents are complex and dynamic, subject to the same shifts and changes as any other relationship. They are determined to a certain extent by cultural factors. In addition, attitudes can change as time passes, so that the same person may see their parents in very different ways as they grow older.

How people with aphasia see their parents

- As a protector.
- As an oppressor.
- As an ally.
- In need of protection and support themselves.

Like others, people who have aphasia may have moved through a number of stages with regards to their feelings about their parents. The onset of language and perhaps physical impairment may mean that they have to return to a previous kind of relationship, one in which they depend upon their parents. Some people feel very comfortable with this. Thus, the independent career woman returns to live with her parents following her stroke and the break-up of her marriage. They create a comfortable and safe environment for her in which she feels protected from the stresses of trying to re-establish work and relationships. She welcomes this support. But others may react to a similar situation with anger:

'My mum is maybe loving me . . . I don't know. Loving as in my child. — But all the time me myself . . . me myself grown up. I don't know. No child. Me grown up but all the time now is the stroke um . . . oh . . . um . . . is . . . oh . . . speaking out. Er . . . is me . . . is angry about Mum. Um . . . little child and cuddle. It's alright . . . but . . .'

Sharon

At the other end of the spectrum, aphasic people may find themselves confronted by the needs of their ageing parents. Communication impairment can become an obstacle to fulfilling this role in a number of ways. Most directly, it can affect the aphasic person's ability to interact with the parent, and to take on an organisational role. Thus the aged parent who has Alzheimer's disease may need clear, simple communication, the very thing which eludes the aphasic son or daughter. Similarly, an elderly parent may need help with making a will or moving into sheltered accommodation, and again the aphasic person may not be able to help with these events. Other factors which can affect the aphasic person's ability to support elderly parents include financial hardship. This can mean that there is not enough money to pay for petrol to go and visit, for example, or, as in one case, that the funeral of a parent cannot be paid for.

Mark's changing relationship with his parents has crossed a wide spectrum of feelings and attitudes. Having relished the freedom of student life, his stroke left him unable to communicate, with significant physical impairments and living at home with his parents, who maintain traditional Hungarian family values. They became very involved in Mark's care and rehabilitation, and now Mark works part-time for his father. He has recently moved to a flat next door to his parents which is *'close, but not too close'*. Mark loves his parents and is grateful to them for all they have done for him, but he sometimes feels hemmed in. He finds it difficult to meet new people and to make new friends. However, he also feels a strong sense of duty towards his parents as they get older. This acts as a motivating force for him: *'I get angry sometimes, sometimes. But my father is different. He listens a hell of a lot but my mother blows up, yeah, blows up. It's the Dynasty or Dallas and what have you. But she calms down afterwards. I also occasionally blows up because of the tension between us. But they are growing old . . . growing old and I want to help her, I want to help them through the difficulties because it's um . . . I really feel it's my . . . my duty. — I got the grit and and from wheelchair person who . . . who I was to what I am today I . . . I owe it. I really feel I owe it to my parents.'*

Mark's account conveys the complexity of his feelings towards his parents. His stroke effectively interrupted the friendships which were so important to him as a student, forcing him to turn back to the home for support and protection.

'All a sudden, they gone. Bye bye': friendships and aphasia

While a degree of support and company may be offered by members of the family, many people have the experience of finding that, following the onset of their aphasia, some of their friendships dwindle and fade away. For better or for worse, families can be held together with tradition and with the rituals of everyday life. Friendships may be equally bound by tradition, but can lack the scaffolding of habit. They are heavily dependent on the use of language, particularly on talking. Friends joke, chat, discuss and advise. Because of the importance of talking in friendship, many aphasic people and their friends find their encounters expose the language impairment before they know how to deal with it. The relationship comes under severe strain and, in many cases, it cracks. This can happen very early on, as friends visit the aphasic person, witness the struggle to communicate and find themselves at a loss as to how to help. They try to deal with the problem by talking a lot themselves, by correcting the aphasic person's attempts to speak, by talking to the partner and not to the aphasic person directly, or by talking in a way which suggests the aphasic person has gone deaf or has become simple-minded:

'They looked at me and looks as if I was very silly. A bit . . . They'd lean over. They'd lean over: "Alright?" I'd say: "I'm not silly." '

Madge

In many cases, friends deal with the situation by abandoning it altogether:

'Just gone. This is it. They gone . . . er . . . about six weeks gone. Gone . . . bye bye. This is it. — I think it's my . . . I can't . . . for a year about six months not communicating really. So they just gone.'

Susan

There are a number of factors which interact and become obstacles to friendship once aphasia becomes established. These are summarised in the box below.

Obstacles to friendship in aphasia

- Changes in work and lifestyle.
- Changes in particular aspects of communication.
- Attitude of friends and of person with aphasia.

Changes in work and lifestyle as an obstacle to friendship

However well-intentioned colleagues may be, it can be hard to maintain social contact with someone who no longer shares the interests and pressures of work which brought them together in the first place. Many aphasic people describe the decline of their social life when they leave work, despite a few visits from friends early on. Losing work can also mean the aphasic person has a restricted income, and this can lead to difficulty meeting the cost of a round of drinks or keeping up a hobby or interest like golf, which had a social component attached.

Other changes, such as lack of mobility, moving house or having to take medication which cannot be combined with alcohol, can mean that the aphasic person is not able to resume old social activities like going to the pub. But lifestyle changes can occur on both sides of the friendship. Some older aphasic people point out that their friends are also becoming elderly and frail, and perhaps less willing to brave a visit after dark. Some outlive old friends. Younger aphasic people may find that their friends start to lose touch as they become caught up in different life events, such as getting married or caring for a young family.

Changes in particular aspects of communication as an obstacle to friendship

Particular aspects of communication can be changed by aphasia, and these can have a rapid and direct effect on the maintenance of friendship. For example, delay in speaking and responding may allow a talkative friend to dominate, determining what is said and how the conversations go, so that the aphasic person feels unable to have any say. The fact that such contact is kindly meant can make it more difficult for the aphasic person to object. Yet it is aggravating and disempowering.

Several people comment that they miss the verbal wit and humour they shared with friends, whether it took the form of quick-fire punning, one-liners or telling jokes and amusing anecdotes. Humorous exchanges are vulnerable when one person has aphasia. This may not be because the person can't think of anything funny to say, but because of the time-lag, as Kiran explains:

'Oh God, my humour was really important. — I used to talk very fast. — I have the humour still but I cannot talk it fast enough. I have to take it in. It goes all the way back into my files and by the time it comes out, it's too late. The conversation has changed. And that is the most . . . hardest thing to accept. I get really, really frustrated when two people are talking and I want to lighten it up with humour. And I cannot do so.'

Some aphasic people miss the long-drawn out, detailed conversations, discussion and debates they used to have with close friends and become reluctant to attempt a contribution which is less profound than they would like. Similarly, those who maintained friendships with letter-writing can find these decline with the onset of aphasia.

> When a stroke left her with quite marked physical impairments, **Janet** and her husband moved to a flat, away from their old friends and neighbours. Her husband cares for Janet at home and although she sometimes gets annoyed if she is rushed, she is very appreciative of his support. She misses seeing her friends, some of whom are now very elderly. But the friendships can't be maintained through writing: *'I haven't had friends because I just haven't been able to write, that's the trouble. My husband will write for me but I mean it's not the same, is it? You can't sort of . . . things that sometimes you like to write and I always write . . . friends, you know . . . I can't do that. I mean it's very good, but there's things we like to write . . . ourselves, don't we? — I think*

> *meself: "I'll just sit down and write a letter and . . ." to my friend and some-body. Can't do it. And then you get you get so frustrated that you won't . . . er . . . then you think "Oh bother it!" — I get so mad with myself.'*

Attitude as an obstacle to friendship

Accounts from this study suggest that aphasia has a profound effect on the dynamics of friendship. The aphasic person may seem to become more passive, more of a recipient than an initiator. However understanding they might be, friends can find this dramatic change difficult to under-stand. When aphasic people talk about friendships which seem to be dwindling, they speculate as to what feelings former friends might have towards them. They suspect that people are impatient, too busy to bother with them, embarrassed or even frightened:

'Thinking about maybe scared with the stroke and speaking out is little bit bad but um . . . scared of what shall I what should . . . what should I say or . . . maybe is muddling with me or . . . I don't know . . . — Made scary of me.'

Sharon

The different nature of friendships between men and those between women is suggested as one explanation for loss of contact.

> *Andrew* was visited by friends from work when he was in hospital following his stroke. He is still angry that one woman friend told his workmates, in his hearing, that he would never walk or speak again. Since his return home, he has lost touch with most of his male friends and has felt ignored: *'They acted as if I wasn't there.'* He puts this down to the competitive nature of their relationship with him and believes that men don't feel comfortable showing concern for some-one who is vulnerable: *'The male friends couldn't talk . . . couldn't do . . . and the er . . . they were sympathetic. I was this . . . you're in the race and you fall over. — It's men because . . . it's er . . . they've got to be there, they can't waste their time worrying about these stroke victims at all. They're not interested, no. — Busy climbing the ladder.'*

Such attitudes obstruct the maintenance of friendships. But they can run both ways. Aphasic people, too, describe feelings of fear, embarrass-ment and shame about their communication which can prevent them from enjoying or initiating contact with friends. For some, the loss of work and other interests makes them feel that they have become dull, and have nothing to contribute to conversation.

Those who are seeking a partner feel aphasia can reduce their chances, both in terms of opportunities to meet new people, and conversations with them, as Mark explains: *'It's very difficult for finding a suitable partner because of my disabilities. — I still er . . . great difficulty communicating because other people are normal. I got to live with that.'*

'I'm fed up of saying I'm sorry': keeping friendships going

People with aphasia react in a number of ways to the threat to their friendships posed by the loss of communication. Some become angry with themselves and with others, some focus on contact with their families, some lose their confidence, become withdrawn and isolated, some feel sad and hurt, but resigned to the situation. But those who do re-establish social contact with friends find they need to develop strategies for dealing with their aphasia.

Strategies for dealing with aphasia in social encounters

- Concealing the aphasia.
- Apologising for the aphasia.
- Integrating the aphasia.
- Being assertive about the aphasia.

Because aphasia cannot be seen, it can remain hidden. A small number of aphasic people, who usually have less marked impairment, find that it is possible to resume the same social life as before, and that difficulties in following or contributing to conversation can be concealed, especially in a large group. Some people find they have to, or wish to acknowledge the aphasia to their friends, but are embarrassed by it, and feel grateful to them for being tolerant. They deal with the aphasia by apologising for it. Occasionally, some find themselves starting to acknowledge the aphasia, talking about it without shame or embarrassment, and feeling comfortable for people to know about it.

Judith was surprised to find herself mentioning stroke and aphasia at a dinner-party, and that people were very interested in what she had to say. She indicates that it was a new experience for her to talk about aphasia in this way, and something she will take time to get used to: '*I say: "I am aphasic." And nobody knows what it is. So I say: "I have speech and language difficulties." It's alright, but it's not a topic I would willingly bring up. I can talk about it now more than I did.*'

Some are able to be assertive about their aphasia. This means telling people about it, and asking them to change or adapt their communication. It might involve arranging to meet friends one-to-one in a quiet place, instead of in a large, noisy group. It might involve asking a friend to repeat, or slow down what they say. It is possible to do this matter-of-factly, explaining the problem and what can be done to help, without apologies and without being aggressive. This sounds easy to do, but it is not:

'*I choose my friends. — I tell them that I got a stroke. I can't speak very well. You got to cope with me.*'

Govi

Those whose friendships and social contact continue as before are outnumbered by those for whom this does not happen. In the long term, many aphasic people face an increasing sense of isolation and exclusion. This is often masked, in the short term, by the fact that the onset of stroke and aphasia brings about other forms of intensive contact, with professionals, volunteers and other people who are 'in the same boat'. Contact with other aphasic people can lead to new networks of friendship, but the early weeks and months of aphasia can be so busy that the changing patterns of social encounters are barely noticed.

5

'Lost in the undertow': health, social care and voluntary services for people with aphasia

The weeks and months following a stroke can be very busy. Both in hospital and back at home, the aphasic person comes into contact with an array of people which can seem overwhelming. Nurses, consultants, housemen, GPs, therapists, social workers, home helps, ambulance drivers, day centre staff, social security personnel, health visitors and volunteers all enter the sphere of the aphasic person, bringing their own concerns and criteria to the encounter, and offering forms of help specific to their own disciplines and backgrounds. The aphasic person does not necessarily expect the needs and problems arising from the stroke to be parcelled out in such a way. Distinctions between services which seem obvious to professionals may not be understood and one service may become mixed up with another. Sorting out who is who and what is offered depends on language which may not be available.

Services experienced by people with aphasia seem to vary widely in terms of their nature, duration, intensity and quality. For example, those taking part in this study spent between five days and fourteen months in hospital. The length of time spent attending out-patient therapies ranged from three months to three and a half years. The intensity of therapies also varied. Some people visited hospital departments as out-patients three or four times a week, others once a fortnight, and others less often, depending on their need and what was available. A few people experienced a seamless transition from hospital to home, as social workers and community-based services efficiently addressed their needs, organising claims for benefits and implementing support in the form of home helps, day centre attendance and household aids and appliances. For others, including two of the youngest respondents who had their strokes most recently, discharge from hospital meant the end of any services. Some continue to have regular contact with stroke clubs and with voluntary and charitable support agencies. Others have never been aware that such services exist. Variations in the type and level of services encountered seem to be in part determined by the severity of the stroke and the nature of the resulting impairments, in part by local policy and availability of resources, and in part by quality and accessibility of information.

In this chapter, the professional and voluntary services experienced by the aphasic people will be described and evaluated in terms of how well they met their changing needs and concerns. Features felt to be characteristic of satisfactory (and unsatisfactory) services will be drawn from the accounts and illustrated. Speech and language therapy services and the role of voluntary and charitable associations will be considered in some detail.

Changing needs and concerns

In the study, the various services encountered were discussed in the context of what aphasic people felt their needs and concerns to be at three different points in time: while they were in hospital; when they first came home; and at the present time.

Type of support required by people with aphasia at three points in time

- *Immediately post-stroke*:
  - medical information, advice and reassurance about the condition;
  - medical treatment, if necessary;
  - treatment, help and advice with physical and communication impairments;
  - help and advice regarding the return home, work and money issues;
  - help with depression and distress;
  - emotional/psychological support;
  - contact with others in similar situation.

- *Coming home*:
  - nursing help and physical assistance, if necessary;
  - aids, equipment and access at home;
  - sorting out the issue of returning to work;
  - help and advice regarding benefits and entitlements;
  - information about local and national services;
  - help with housework;

– medical information and advice;
– contact with, reassurance and information from GP;
– support for care-givers;
– assistance with transport;
– help with depression and distress;
– emotional/psychological support for self and family;
– continuing treatment for and advice about physical and
  communication impairments;
– contact with others in similar situation;
– access to educational and leisure opportunities.

- *Five years and more post-stroke*:
  – flexible support, for example, when care-giver becomes ill;
  – help with rehousing;
  – regular medical checks, reassurance and advice;
  – information about local health, social care and voluntary services;
  – contact and reassurance regarding physical and
    communication impairments;
  – help with financial problems;
  – help with continuing depression and distress;
  – support for care-givers;
  – physical aids and assistance if necessary;
  – access to educational and leisure opportunities;
  – access to national voluntary and charitable associations;
  – contact with others in similar situation.

Some sorts of support seem to be required consistently both in the early days and years after the stroke. Thus, for many, a desire for contact with others in a similar situation persists for years following the stroke. But it is also possible to discern shifts in focus as time passes. Early on, people describe acute concern about the medical aspects of the stroke and a desire for treatment to improve the resulting impairments. Later, this becomes overshadowed by a need for on-going contact, reassurance and support regarding the impairments, information about services, and concern about practical issues such as sorting out financial, domestic and work problems.

While the list shows the broad patterns of concern, it does not convey the range of different attitudes towards seeking and accepting support from professional and voluntary services. For example, some who experience financial hardship in the aftermath of stroke are unwilling to seek help by claiming benefits because they see this as accepting charity or scrounging off the state. Some see social services support in their home as a potential threat to their privacy and independence. Emotional distress is seen by some as a form of moral weakness, better resolved by pulling one-self together and gritting one's teeth than by finding help in the form of counselling. In addition, it seems that the attitudes of individual people towards using services can change as time passes. For example, some people recall high levels of emotional distress in the days and weeks following their stroke. Although at the time they would have welcomed some kind of support, such as counselling, they now feel that they have coped for many years without it. To seek help at this point would be to suggest failure and defeat.

What makes a service satisfactory?

Many of the aphasic people who took part in this study had some experi-ence of services which were adequate and appropriate to their particular needs and with which they were satisfied. Indeed, most are appreciative of those who provide services and aware of the pressures under which they operate. Drawing on the detailed accounts of the people who took part in this study, it is possible to piece together recipients' views of the features which characterise successful service provision. These may not correspond with the views of those who plan, provide and manage ser-vices.

Attributes of successful services

- Availability and accessibility.
- Appropriateness and adequacy.
- Flexibility and responsiveness.
- Integration.
- Reliability and consistency.
- Respectfulness.
- Able to support communication.
- Providing relevant and accessible information.

Availability and accessibility

An available service is one which is provided to meet a particular need, for example, the need for emotional support, for information about aphasia or for help with household tasks. In order to take advantage of such a service, the potential recipient needs to be aware that it exists and how to use it. Available services should also be accessible. It is usual to think of access in physical terms, as something which can be provided by building ramps, widening doorways and providing toilets which it is possible for wheelchair-users to enter. Of course, many aphasic people who have physical impairments do need services to be physically accessible.

But people with aphasia also need communicative access to services. Those who are able to understand what services are available, to make a phone call, to explain what they want to a secretary or receptionist, to follow up a name and number given out in the hospital or jotted down from a poster, to fix appointments and note them down, to write a letter requesting prompt action, may be able to improve, increase or speed up access to the services they receive. Aphasia can obstruct these seemingly commonplace processes with the result that access to the service becomes blocked.

Appropriateness and adequacy

In the view of people with aphasia, services need to be both appropriate and adequate. Appropriate services are those which are relevant to the needs and requirements of the individual, offering support which is useful and useable at a particular point in time. Those who take up services and those who provide them may have different views about the appropriateness of services. But the issue of whether or not a service is adequate will almost certainly lead to disagreement. A commonly expressed view concerns the desire for more prolonged contact with therapists and other professionals. What seems to be required is not so much continuous treatment, but ongoing reassurance, advice and support.

Timeliness and flexibility

A satisfactory service, in the view of people with aphasia, is one which is promptly delivered at the appropriate time and which is nevertheless flexible in responding to their changing needs.

Integration

A satisfactory service is seen to be one which addresses changing needs in an integrated way, taking on the real-life problems which occur, and based on understanding the person as a complex social being, rather than as an isolated set of impairments. Related to this, many of the aphasic people who took part in this study comment on their wish for a degree of integration between hospital and community-based services, a sense of being 'followed up'. Being discharged from hospital can lead to feelings of being abandoned and pushed aside for those who are not contacted once they return home.

Reliability and consistency

For people with aphasia, constantly changing or tentative arrangements can be difficult to understand and to retain unless they are carefully explained and recorded in a way which can be understood. Rules, regulations and arrangements need to be clear and consistent. It is important that the same person consistently follows up contact, because it can take time for those who have no language impairment to understand what aphasia is and to get to know the aphasic person's style of communicating. Another commonly reported inconsistency which causes difficulty for aphasic people concerns the way in which some professionals and officials reach decisions about eligibility for and provision of suitable services. This process can run smoothly and efficiently but often decisions are made, contested and reversed. Thus, a GP and a consultant may disagree about the most appropriate dosage of a medication and will give the aphasic person contradictory instructions. Some people describe the bewildering effect of inconsistent responses to their applications for particular benefits, aids and appliances. Some accounts describe a succession of officers reaching different and contradictory conclusions about one person's eligibility for a particular benefit or appliance. The uncertainty arising from such contradictions can be unsettling for someone who has aphasia. Like others, those who have aphasia wish their concerns to be met with clear and consistent decisions.

The reliability of a service is also important to people who have aphasia. Aphasia makes it difficult to understand tentative arrangements, to ring up and enquire about what has happened if a promised service does not appear, and to request further contact. Therefore appointments need to be clearly arranged, to be definite and to be kept, if at all possible. If there is a problem, it is important that the aphasic person is informed, and understands any new arrangements.

Respect and acknowledgement

Difficulty communicating can be worsened by the rushed and busy approach which seems characteristic of many in the caring professions. Aphasic people appreciate the pressure under which many professionals are working, but describe how the 'busy-ness' of doctors, therapists, social security personnel and others makes them feel that they are holding these important people up.

Even though in some cases the ability to understand the content and detail of what is being said may be limited, people with aphasia are extremely sensitive to the tone of the speaker and the attitude which is being conveyed. Although they may not be able to challenge or object to negative attitudes they encounter, aphasic people may rightly feel a sense of anger if they are not treated with respect.

Supporting communication

When negotiating or receiving a service, people who have aphasia benefit from any effort to support their communication. Essentially, this means that the person providing a service needs to give the exchange time, checking with the aphasic person what can be done to make communication easier, as different strategies may be useful for different people. Commonly used strategies which can help the person who has aphasia to understand involve talking slowly and backing up speech with writing. Strategies useful in supporting the aphasic person's expression of their wishes, needs and concerns involve encouraging the use of writing, drawing and gesture, if speech is a problem. It is also important that the non-aphasic person constantly checks and reverifies what has been established by reviewing the conversation at regular intervals. But those who provide services for people with aphasia may be unfamiliar with language impairment, uncertain what it means and unsure how to approach it. In addition, they may not be able or willing to change their styles of communication, or even aware that this is necessary. The individual needs of aphasic people complicate the demands upon the non-aphasic speaker.

Providing relevant and accessible information

For aphasic people, the very tools needed for finding, understanding and using information are damaged. This means that information needs to be brought to the aphasic person's attention, and made available in an accessible form.

These perceptions of what constitutes successful and satisfactory services are relevant to all those working in health and social care. They cut across professional and institutional boundaries. In Figure 5.1, some examples of positive and negative experiences of a range of different services will be listed under each of the attributes described.

Figure 5.1 The experience of services

POSITIVE EXPERIENCES	NEGATIVE EXPERIENCES
1 Availability and accessibility	
Health care	
– Regular visits from GP	– Hours spent waiting for transport to therapy
– Local clinic runs health checks	– Therapy in first language not available
Social care and support	
– Help with the household arranged	– Distress not acknowledged or helped

POSITIVE EXPERIENCES	NEGATIVE EXPERIENCES
– Proactive support from social worker	– Social services never answer phone
Social security	
– Support filling in forms	– Unable to understand leaflets + forms
	– Standing for hours in DSS office queue

'In the early stages, it would have meant a lot to me if I could have talked to somebody as I've talked to you.'

Geoffrey

'I am phoning social services. Ring ring. No answer. Four times. Four times. No answer. No, no, no. The social services — no — forget it.'

Robert

2 Appropriateness and adequacy

Health care

– Follow-up appointments with consultant	– Irrelevant therapy + day-care activities
– Contact with therapists over years	– Placement in unsuitable group or ward

Social care and support

– Suitable aids + adaptations arranged	– Social worker never appears
	– Day Centre does not provide help with bathing

Social security

– Adequate financial support to live independently	– Benefits and entitlements never arranged: prolonged hardship, poverty and anxiety

'I haven't had sufficient therapy.'

Ted

'We got the impression they hadn't got the staff.'

Jean

3 Timeliness and flexibility

Health care

– Appointments with GP promptly arranged	– Waiting months for therapy

Social care and support

– Home support sorted out before discharge	– Years for handrail to be provided

Social security

	– Seven years before benefits shortfall noticed

'After a few years I managed to get the doctor from Social Security to come and see me and then I got the pension.'

Martha

'It took years to get that handrail down there.'

Tom

POSITIVE EXPERIENCES	NEGATIVE EXPERIENCES

4 Carry-over from hospital to community

Health care

– Outpatient follow-up arranged
– Home visits from therapists before
  discharge
	– Complete cessation of services
	  and contact on discharge

Social care and support
– Social worker continues contact	– No support on discharge

Social security
	– No idea of existence of benefits

'The worst thing that ever happened to me was no follow-up. None at all from then to this day.'

Fred

'No check to see how your ticker is or your brain. How's your brain. You're a forgotten person'

Tom

5 Reliability and consistency

Health care
– Continuous contact with one person – Knowing who to contact	– A new doctor at every consultation – GP and consultant keep changing medication

Social care and support

– Being given the name and phone
  number of a social worker
– Same home help comes every day
	– Social worker makes vague arrange-
	  ment to call and doesn't turn up
	– Home help withdrawn without
	  explanation

Social security
	– Contradictory decisions on eligibility

'Switch on the telly, there is a new rule.'

Ravi

'She said: "See you next week" and I didn't see her no more.'

Bert

6 Respect and acknowledgement

Health care

– GP listens to and tries to address
  problems
	– Houseman seems patronising, makes
	  jokes about impairment, busy and
	  rushed
	– Therapist bossy and irritable

Social care and support

– Aphasic person consulted in change
  of arrangements
	– Social worker fails to keep
	  appointments

POSITIVE EXPERIENCES	NEGATIVE EXPERIENCES
Social security	
– Social worker acts as advocate	– High-handed manner of DSS staff
	– Staff work 9–5. No concern

'The doctors, the doctors. — Yeah . . . I hate . . . yeah I hate er . . . patronising. — It's sort of offish and I'm the boss.'

Mark

'They talked to my wife. It doesn't help if she is white. Ignoring me because I am black and also because I was ill.'

Kiran

7 Communication

Health care	
– Consultant draws diagram to explain stroke	– Consultant talks too quickly
	– GP looks at notes when talking
Social care and support	
– Home help gives time to communication	
– Social worker familiar with what helps communication, gives time	
Social security	
	– Official rushed and irritable

'They're talking to their notes and not to you.'

Mike

8 Information

Health care	
– Consultant uses analogy to explain blood flow	– Not warned about fits
– Nurse explains outlook	– No explanation of aphasia given
Social care and support	
– Range of options explained	– No idea of what aids are available
– Information + advice given at Day Centre	– Not told about taxi card, holiday scheme, bus pass, disabled badge for car
Social security	
– Social worker guides and supports claim	– No idea who to ask for advice
	– Frustrated + harassed staff have no time

'Speak and phone . . . no I can't. So, you know, who advise? Hospital . . . nothing, nothing.'

Cath

Two examples of the experience of services

Although it is rare to find wholly positive or wholly negative accounts across the spectrum of health, social care and other services, the following accounts show the extent to which aphasic people's experience can vary. Madge feels that she has been supported and that the care she has received has been satisfactory. Rebecca's views are very different.

Madge is generally satisfied with the way health and social services have worked for her since her stroke. Despite her significant physical impairment and aphasia, Madge wanted to return to living independently at home: *'It was through the social worker in the hospital. She was very kind and she sorted everything out for me. Before I came out of the hospital it was arranged I would have a home help. They had a meeting, and I was able to have them every day. Every day. Seven days a week.'* Madge's speech is very indistinct, but her regular home help has got to know her well and is now able to understand most of what she says. She has also developed strategies to use when she cannot understand, for example, sitting down with Madge in a relaxed way and giving her full attention to the conversation. Madge values this long-term support. As well as organising the home-help service, the social worker arranged for Madge to attend a day centre and local stroke club, and even to have a holiday. Through the occupational therapy services, she has been provided with a stair-lift and other aids and appliances in the house: *'I'm full of praise. There's nothing too much. Everything I've wanted I've had.'* Despite her generally positive feelings about her own experience, Madge is aware that others are not so well-served. She feels that she has perhaps been able to pull strings, because she knew people in the social work and occupational therapy departments through her previous work. She also points out that it took a friend to tell her about the Independent Living Fund, for which she successfully applied. Without this money, which she uses to employ extra assistance, she would not be so comfortable: *'The social services are very good, but it's not good enough.'* Madge is also critical of the social services day centre she attended, because of the length of time she had to wait before she could have a bath there. If Madge needs help or advice, she has the names and numbers of those in the occupational therapy and social work services to whom she would turn and who know her well.

Rebecca's experience of health and other services has made her angry. When she had her stroke, she was taken to hospital, where, after some delay because it was a bank holiday, she underwent various tests. Initially, there was some uncertainty about what might be causing her physical weakness and her inability to express what she wanted to say: *'One of the doctors said to me: "This doesn't happen to 22-year-old girls and we're not used to dealing with it."'* Rebecca was referred to a psychiatrist, confirming her fear that she was going mad: *'They just said to me: "Oh it's all in your head, all in your mind"* — *They treated me like an idiot. They're so sort of condescending. I mean they wouldn't talk to me like that now because I'm . . . you know I can communicate. But when you can't communicate, they treat you like a kid and that is just so frustrating.* — *A handful of the doctors were just awful. You just wanted to say: "Do you know what this is like?"* Rebecca tried to convey the fact that her field of vision was impaired to one doctor: *'He said: "Explain what you mean" and of course I couldn't and he sat there sort of tapping his fingers. He said: "Well does that mean you can't see countryside?" I said . . . I just thought . . . I just didn't bother.'* Although she had intensive treatment from physiotherapists who were *'like Rottweilers'*, Rebecca had no contact with a speech and language therapist, despite her impaired communication: *'It was never even offered. It was never an option.'* On her discharge from hospital she had no information about services, no follow-up from her GP, no contact with an occupational therapist or social worker, and had no idea of the existence of support agencies and local groups. While she appreciates that those in the caring professions are overstretched, Rebecca still feels devalued by her hospital experience. She wanted: *'For somebody just to commit themselves and said what . . . just to come up to me and say: "This is what's happened to you and this is what we're going to . . . this is what'll . . ." You know, because there was nothing. It was all just up in the air and I got round it in my own way* — *It makes me very angry the way I was treated, specially being so young.* — *It's just the disregard they had for people with strokes. Not only me, it's just the whole . . . the whole thing. They just sort of cart you off and give you wheelchairs. Thank you very much. Next!* — *These people are forgotten about.'*

'You can't make yourself known': aphasia and negotiation

Many non-aphasic people experience similar problems with health, social and other services to those described in this chapter. However, people who have a communication impairment become particularly vulnerable.

Aphasia makes it difficult to enquire, to understand, to query, to negotiate services and to object. Often, because aphasia cannot be seen, its
nature and effects are not understood and the vulnerability of those who
are struggling to communicate is not perceived. This may mean that they
go without services which would be useful to them. For many aphasic
people, loss of language means a loss of control over what is happening.

Elderly and physically frail, *Martha* lives alone and is dependent
upon the support of a home help and district nurses. Martha worked
as a doctor and she is not impressed with her experience of being on
the receiving end of services. From her perspective, it seems that the
medical profession have little understanding of aphasia: *'They don't
necessarily know what it means.'* She is critical of the services she
experiences and blames cutbacks in health resources. Her main complaints concern the lack of time she is given in consultations with her
GP, and a home-nursing service which seems to have been honed
down: *'First of all they're not enough and then she'll ring up and says sorry
she can't come this week and I mean I won't be washed for two weeks. I've
just had an ulcer on there. I've had it now for ages but nobody has looked at
it for two weeks, have they? They're awful.'* While Martha has threatened
to complain about the dwindling services she has received, she is
aware that she would have difficulty carrying this out: *'I told them that
if they . . . if they . . . if they . . . I've forgotten what it was about now. I said
I was writing to the Prime Minister about this . . . oh very blasé. — I would
take all day about it . . . if about . . . and do it and do it . . . — Mmm, mm.
And write it again and again and again until I . . .'* Martha has found a
way round her problem communicating with doctors who cannot
give her enough time. She pays for private treatment: *'My physician is
particularly good. I knew him personally and he takes my whole thing up. He
looks me whole, whole body, the whole body. — He's an awfully nice person
anyway. He's very quiet and peaceful and when I go . . . if I getting, you
know, stuck he'll say: "Now wait a minute, we'll go back to the beginning
and we'll start again." — That's why he's not a National Health doctor.'*

In some cases, aphasic people express the feeling that perhaps they have
been more useful to, than helped by, some of the services. One man contributed to a speech and language therapy research project by sitting
through many hours of testing and experimentation. He never understood the purpose or the outcome of the study. The therapist had no
further contact with him once his part in the project came to an end.
Another had the experience of being used on a regular basis to demon-
strate aphasia to large groups of medical students:

'They had a area . . . area for students . . . all these . . . theatres and asking me things and er . . . at that time I was having trouble with um . . . things with with . . . er names of um . . . oh like these. Like oh . . . you've seen this and er . . . I would push something else. — When I found out that I was doing it, I should be doing this and I was doing that, then I thought I was stupid.'

Rob

While both of these people were compliant and good-natured in contributing to teaching and research, the fact that they were doing so with compromised language raises some important questions about the issue of informed consent. Aphasia may make it difficult to understand the purpose and nature of professional activities and to make a truly informed decision about taking part.

It is possible too for those who have aphasia to find solutions to the problems encountered in accessing and using services, but this largely depends on harnessing the goodwill of others. In some cases, friends and family fill the gaps in the provision of physical care and support. Some also take on the often protracted and frustrating task of sorting out benefits, arranging therapy and negotiating the installation of aids and appliances. Some aphasic people locate particular professionals and stick to them, teaching them about their aphasia and effectively using them as advocates to whom they turn whenever they encounter problems. And some who are able to do so simply pay for services which are not generally available, and for more or better quality professional time.

'I must be daft': experiences of speech and language therapy

The experiences described in this chapter concern a number of different services, medical, financial, social, therapeutic and community-based. The attributes drawn from these accounts are therefore relevant to all of those who provide care for aphasic people, from consultants to home helps, from social workers to social security personnel. In looking more closely at one particular service (speech and language therapy), it is possible to develop a more detailed understanding of each of the attributes and features which aphasic people feel to be important and to consider the implications for the professionals involved.

Speech and language therapy is a complex service which should be particularly relevant to anybody who has aphasia. It comprises a number of processes, including assessment of the language impairment, advice and, if appropriate, treatment by a qualified therapist. At the time of writing, in the UK, an open system of referral is used. This means that anyone, including the aphasic person, can make a referral to the therapist.

However, the rise of independently run healthcare trusts means that local policies on referral and management of people who have aphasia may start to differ throughout the country.

Availability and accessibility of speech and language therapy

The availability of a speech and language therapy service for people with aphasia seems to vary widely from region to region with the result that some people have years of contact with a speech and language therapist and others, like Rebecca, are never referred for therapy at all. Some people are simply not aware that it might be an option. Of people who are referred, those who have a similar type and severity of aphasia can receive widely varying amounts and types of therapy.

Knowing that a service is available but being unable to access it can prove intensely frustrating for the aphasic person who is desperate for help and advice:

Betty was discharged from hospital, physically able but with a marked aphasia. She is still angry about the fact that she was left to cope with her aphasia alone and was never followed up by the speech therapy service: *'The speech therapist came once or twice and gave me one of those tests, you know, with the spelling and everything and I couldn't make head nor tail of it. — She came, I think a week later and suggested I had a speech therapist. But they were a bit short at the time. That was a bit awful, but they never phoned . . . followed it up and I said, bravely you know: "I can manage without." — I had visited the hospital to the specialist three times and that was it. She said: "Oh well, I think you're the type who can do it yourself." Well my cousins brought me home and brought me to the supermarket because . . . so as to get things. Afterwards my next door neighbour went up to bring me things. But apart from that nobody knew. Everybody thought I was alright. — I was a bit peeved about the speech because I realised I wanted . . . I needed it. I still do, of course. I do resent not having the speech therapist.'*
Access to therapy, in Betty's case, seems to have been blocked by limited resources and by the failure of those providing services to perceive her need for help and support. Betty herself shied away from pushing for provision, partly because she had little faith in her language at the time.

Physical access to speech and language therapy can also be a problem in terms of transport to and from the sessions. The aphasic person who is unable to drive may spend hours waiting for and riding around on an ambulance, in order to receive forty minutes of therapy. Those who have braved public transport to get to therapy describe the difficulties of asking a driver for a busfare and fumbling for change in a queue of impatient people. Such experiences are often felt to outweigh any benefits of therapy.

The nature and appropriateness of speech and language therapy

When asked about what speech and language therapy entails, people who have aphasia describe a number of different activities. These include exercises for tongue and facial muscles, practice producing the sounds of speech, exercises on grouping words together according to their meanings, work on using and understanding grammatical structures, reading and writing exercises and group discussions. Most people understand the purpose of therapy sessions as being some kind of retraining or reactivation of their language. However, a small number find themselves mystified by the type of thing they were asked to do in therapy. The purpose of activities such as naming or describing pictures of objects or events, used by therapists to gather information about the type and severity of the aphasia, is sometimes not understood. Some therapists seem to be poor at conveying information about what is being done in therapy, and why. As a result, to some aphasic people the rituals of therapy seem demeaning and make them feel stupid. Many people point out that therapy can feel like returning to the classroom. The association with school can sometimes be reinforced by the manner of the therapist:

'It was cat and dog and all that. I had to try and do a cat and another cat. I didn't know why but I do now. — I must be daft . . . something like that. But the speech therapy know best sort of thing.'

Philip

Despite this, many of those who experienced speech and language therapy, including those who did not understand the purpose of particular activities, see it as having had a positive effect in helping to sort out their difficulties:

'He had me making sounds. Phonetic sound. It helps you speak. — He straightened it out. — I got on very well.'

Les

As well as helping to restore language, therapy is appreciated because it increases confidence in communication and can bring the aphasic person into contact with others in a similar situation. A small number of people enjoyed the services of speech and language therapists who seemed to be concerned, not only with their language impairment but with their general well-being. Such therapists seem to have addressed issues beyond the language impairment, for example setting up contact with other agencies such as counsellors and adult education classes, enlisting the help of social workers, introducing the aphasic person to self-help groups and organising other services such as aphasia-friendly assertiveness training. However, other accounts of speech and language therapy suggest it can be totally irrelevant to the needs and concerns of aphasic people. Such disparate experiences, of the availability, amount and quality of therapy suggest a fundamental inequity of service:

Rose and **Kiran**, who had similar strokes within two years of each other, resulting in similar impairments, had very different experiences of speech and language therapy. Rose had a brief encounter with a therapist in hospital when she first lost her language, but did not find what was offered helpful or appropriate: *'I got visited by the speech therapist and she did, like cards that said "yes" and "no" and all the things that I like to eat and drink. I took them gratefully but I couldn't read them and I couldn't explain to her that I couldn't read them so I just took them, thinking: "Oh she'll go away in a minute."'* Rose was not followed up when she was discharged home to look after her two young children, even though she had virtually no language at that point. Although she lives in a rural setting, Rose was within striking distance of a large conurbation, and could have attended out-patient therapy there, had any been arranged: *'It was disgusting. They kept telling me that somebody would come out but they never came so that really was the total speech therapy I got. I think so much more money ought to be provided for these follow-up services.'* In contrast, Kiran had twice-weekly contact with a therapist while he was in hospital and regular out-patient appointments for six months after he came home. He feels the speech and language therapy he received was critically important for his recovery. Although both he and his therapist wished to continue therapy beyond the six month limit (*'. . . recovery can go on for a long, long time . . .'*) he understood that the pressure of the waiting list meant he had to be discharged. His therapist worked on his language impairment, and also provided some basic counselling. Together they put forward a successful case for developing a post for a Panjabi-speaking therapist. Despite their different experiences, Kiran and Rose both feel that they would have benefited from more speech and language therapy.

Adequacy of speech and language therapy

Individual contact with a speech and language therapist can continue for years. Some people who took part in this study are still attending communication groups run by therapists up to nine years after their stroke.

Others continue to attend self-help groups and stroke clubs, some of which are supported by therapists. This prolonged contact stands in marked contrast to the experience of those who have had minimal contact with the service.

Most criticisms of the speech and language therapy service concern the fact that people think they haven't had enough of it. If they could, many would still be continuing with therapy even years after the stroke. This seems to be either because they believe therapy could bring more of their language back or because they feel their abilities are increasing anyway but they are in need of advice and reassurance as they progress.

'I think two hours or three hours a week needed.'

Colin

Interviewer: Do you think that helped you at all, the speech therapy?
Jack: Oh no . . . one week.
Interviewer: One week?
Jack: Yeah . . . well. Once . . . a . . . week
Interviewer: Once a week. Do you think that's enough, Jack?
Jack: (angry) Oh bloody hell!
Interviewer: Not at all.
Jack: One two three four five.
Interviewer: It should be four times a week or . . .
Jack: Yeah. Bloody hell. Oh bloody hell.

The attitude and communication skills of speech and language therapists

Speech and language therapists generally seem to be appreciated by people with aphasia. Their skills in facilitating communication and in offering emotional support, the fact that they seem to understand what aphasia is, and their acknowledgement of the aphasic person are all met with relief, perhaps because these attributes seem rarely encountered elsewhere. The anxiety which is focused on the aphasia, together with the hope that this person will be able to improve the situation, can lead to some intense feelings towards the therapist which often overlay memories of previous 'teachers'. The power of the therapist in this relationship can be considerable. Those who are high-handed, dismissive, bossy or antagonistic towards their aphasic clients can have a devastating impact. Nevertheless, anger at the inadequacies of therapy is rarely directed at the therapist, rather levelled at those who organise and manage health services, and at politicians:

'The Tory Govern . . . is not much money'

Stephen

'I want to bang their heads together. I want to fight for aphasia therapy.'

Kiran

'There's insufficient funds given by the government.'

Alf

Information, integration and the ending of therapy

The ending of therapy can be very significant for the person with aphasia. It may be the point at which the long-term nature of the aphasia is faced, highlighted by the knowledge that there will be no further direct work on promoting recovery. At this point, too, the aphasic person may need different types of information: about the aphasia, whether further recovery is likely, and what local resources might be called upon. However, as well as being poor at giving information about the nature of aphasia and the purpose of therapy, some speech and language therapists seem to have difficulty explaining why therapy is ending, what the outlook is and what the options are.

Ways in which therapy was ended

- Finished abruptly: *'It just seemed to cut dead.'*
- Discontinued with some explanation: *'I was up to a certain point. I could read a bit. I could talk and she said can't afford to keep me on.'*
- Tailed off gradually: *'It was stages, stages.'*
- Negotiated and planned: *'We discuss when we go out.'*

Reasons for therapy coming to an end

- No reason given: *'They cancelled that. Why I don't know, but they did.'*
- Limited resources: *'I had to make room for the next person.'*
- Further therapy unlikely to be helpful: *'They told me they can't do any more.'*
- Aphasic person wants to stop: *'I felt they were wasting their time.'*
- Therapist stops work: *'He left his job.'*

Therapy can be ended in a number of different ways and for a number of different reasons. Although they understand that services are rationed, many people describe being upset at the way their therapy ended, especially if this happened abruptly and with no explanation. The preferred method is a gradual easing off of contact, coupled with careful explanation, together with discussion of options and ways of coping with real-life problems. The fact that this rarely happens suggests that speech and language therapists may have difficulty integrating aphasia therapy with the real-life issues faced by people with aphasia. Some accounts suggest a sense of speech and language therapy being remote from the real concerns of the person who is trying to live with aphasia:

Vincent's language skills were assessed by a speech and language therapist when he first had a stroke. He was shocked by the apparent simplicity of the things he was asked to do and his inability to do them: *'She put some little things like a penny and a cup and a spoon. And she would say to me: "Look on the wall there, what is that?" And I when she saying it, deep down I thought, well I'm stupid, you know? But then when I look I can't . . . I can't visualise what she's saying — So I find . . . oh it was worse than ever I thought.'* Following his discharge from hospital, Vincent had some individual therapy and then moved onto group sessions. Vincent is full of admiration for the speech and language therapists he met, whom he felt were working under pressure in cramped and difficult conditions: *'I think they deserve a medal. I get a lot of benefit from it. I think I really gain a lot of experience with the different than people with stroke.'* Weekly group therapy involved quizzes and language games. At the time he was consumed with a desire to return to work and was extremely anxious about his financial and home situation. While not being at all critical, Vincent points out that the weekly activities in speech and language therapy did not touch on these issues: *'I personally had got a bit bored. — I learned a lot of things that I didn't know when I had the stroke, like the history of the Royals. — The speech therapy didn't give me information about help. The help they give me is to try and get better.'* Vincent eventually left the group, but stays in touch with some of the people he met there.

'I suppose I have to enjoy it': the role of the voluntary sector

As well as describing their experience of services, the aphasic people who took part in this study also talked about their contact with various voluntary and charitable associations. The main national charitable organisations offering help and support to people with aphasia in the UK are the Stroke Association (which has set up national network of Dysphasia Support language groups across the country, run by trained volunteers) and Action for Dysphasic Adults (which has helped to establish and support a number of regional social and self-help groups). Both organisations supply information and advice about aphasia. ADA (Action for Dysphasic Adults) is in the process of developing an extensive range of initiatives, including training programmes for medical students and residential care staff, expert witness support for aphasic people involved in legal proceedings and aphasia-friendly information about specific language impairments and the nature of therapies. Both ADA and the Stroke Association seek to work in co-operation with speech and language therapy services. In addition to the national charitable organisations, some regions are served by local charitable foundations and by voluntary services which run local stroke clubs and stroke groups, sometimes with the involvement of a speech and language therapist.

The types of voluntary and charitable services encountered by aphasic people in this study are summarised in the box below.

Voluntary and charitable services encountered by people with aphasia

- Information from national charitable organisations such as Action for Dysphasic Adults (ADA) and the Stroke Association (SA).
- Membership of regional social groups set up and supported by ADA.
- Membership of self-help groups supported by ADA.
- Membership of local Dysphasia Support language groups set up by the SA.
- Use of items such as 'communication cards' explaining aphasia to members of the public, supplied by ADA and SA.
- Membership of stroke clubs supported and run by volunteers, organised by local charitable bodies in conjunction with local health services.
- Contact with other voluntary services such as the Citizens' Advice Bureaux.
- Regular visits from volunteers organised locally by charities and health services.

As with statutory services, the extent and nature of aphasic people's contact with the voluntary sector varies widely, depending largely on what is available and personal preference. Some people have no contact at all with voluntary bodies and no idea that they exist. Some make little use of the services which are available to them. Others devote considerable time each week to attending meetings and groups. Attitudes to such services also vary widely. For some, the support and contact is invaluable and the work done by the organisations assumes a central importance. Some who join groups, particularly self-help groups, rediscover their ability to be dynamic in social interactions. Others are happy to find themselves in a position in which they are the recipients of care, sympathy and support.

What aspects of voluntary and charitable services are valued?

Aphasic people value three main aspects of voluntary and charitable services. First, many people make the point that the clubs, groups and contacts supported by voluntary and charitable organisations give the opportunity to meet others who are 'in the same boat', to make friends, to share experiences, and to acquire information and advice with and from other people who are going through the same experience. Secondly, many accounts suggest that the clubs and groups are 'safe havens'. Aphasic people feel that their communication problems are understood and accepted. They do not stand out and have a respite from feelings of social exclusion. Many describe the positive effect of such contact on their levels of confidence. Thirdly, some people have found the charitable and voluntary organisations to be a useful source of much-needed information and advice.

Voluntary services: expectations of people with aphasia

- Information about the service which is accessible ('aphasia-friendly') and available early on.
- Accessible local service.
- Contact with others with aphasia through voluntary visiting scheme to be available immediately post-stroke.
- Education and training about aphasia for others, especially those providing health and social services.
- Effective help and support for the aphasic person dealing with financial, personal, legal and social problems.
- The possibility of choosing different types of contact with others, for example in social, 'therapy'-based and self-help groups.

What problems do people perceive with voluntary and charitable services?

While expressing their appreciation, aphasic people have three main concerns about their experience of services provided by voluntary and charitable bodies. First, not everyone gets to hear about what they do and how to access their services. Secondly, some services are felt to be inadequate in the sense that they do not address the day to day problems encountered by aphasic people, for example difficulty getting benefits sorted out or getting access to social services support:

'There's nobody . . . even now . . . nobody . . . nobody . . . no-one to tell the people up our club what they're entitled to . . . regarding their money. No-one at all. I mean . . . I tell them all. — Our warden up at the club . . . well she's a big help but she's not the help she should be. I told her. I said: "You're not helping people by explaining what they're entitled to." I would have thought they would have done that. — They ought to know their job properly.'

Fred

Thirdly, although meeting others in the same situation can be a liberating experience, it is also possible to feel uncomfortable being associated with groups of people with similar disabilities. For some, especially younger people, being 'placed' in a group of people with disabilities and becoming the recipient of organised care comes as an unwelcome shock. Some aphasic people resolve this problem by taking on the role of 'helper' to the others. But the stress caused by the damage to their self-image can lead some aphasic people to stop attending, or simply tolerate the meetings because of the lack of alternatives:

Having left hospital and finished speech and language therapy, *Govi* had some contact with the Stroke Association. A volunteer visitor was organised to help him with reading and writing, and he made extensive use of the Stroke Association card explaining aphasia, especially early on, when he was struggling to communicate. In the first few months after his discharge from therapy, Govi was pleased to attend a Dysphasia Support group. He speaks warmly of the group organiser: *'She was a very nice girl. I was very appreciated her.'* Govi valued meeting other people with aphasia: *'I feel sorry for them. They feel sorry for me also. — Nice to know them. And because that moment was very nice alright . . . when I go. They welcome you. And she is very good. Er . . . variety of programme with one day.'* However, his feelings gradually changed: *'For the start. And everyone when you got a stroke that started very nice. — I not complaining one bit. No, no. Is after that when you're er . . . I mean when you want to be independent. Alright? You want to do your own things, I mean. Then is bad. — If you never do other things, you're gone with the wind. — Different people. I think so, they want to go there. For they happy. They are happy there. They want to go every day if possible. I'm sorry to say I'm a different person I want to be independence.'* Govi stopped attending, although he still keeps in touch with the organiser.

Their accounts suggest that aphasic people have high expectations of voluntary as well as health and social care services. These can be summarised in three main ways. First, they require that their needs are acknowledged and that some attempt is made to meet these in an appropriate way as they change over the weeks, months and years following the stroke. Secondly, they require those who provide services to acknowledge their situation, to make efforts to support their communication and to treat them with respect. Thirdly, they require information on relevant issues to be given in the right form and at the right time. These requirements apply to all those who offer services, from home help to GP, social security officer to consultant. They concern all aspects of the services offered, from organisation to attitude.

Others who have a long-lasting illness or condition may share the expectations and experiences of various services described in this chapter. But their language impairment places those who have aphasia at a particular disadvantage. It reduces their control over what is happening. Unable to make themselves known, their vulnerability is often not apparent to those who are planning and providing services.

6

'Everything seems a secret':
information and aphasia

Information comes in many forms. It can be acquired through reading leaflets, books, advertisements and posters, through TV, radio and computer networks, through talking with professionals, friends and acquaintances. In order to track down the information needed in any particular situation it may be necessary to jot down a phone number or an address, fill in a form, write a letter, make a call to enquire about a service or to ask for an explanation. All these activities involve language. Like other people, those who have aphasia require information, but the nature of their impairment can mean that their access to it is blocked. The process of locating, selecting and understanding information depends on the very skills which have been weakened. In this chapter, the information needs of aphasic people will be traced through the immediate aftermath of stroke and in the longer term. Different views of the importance of information will be described. Particular problems and possible solutions will be outlined.

'I still don't understand what wrong with me': the information needs of aphasic people

The information needs of people with aphasia can change as time passes. Concerns about life and death issues, such as survival or the likelihood of another stroke are always present, but perhaps are less intensely felt as the months pass and confidence gradually returns. As the aphasic person becomes more familiar with the impairments resulting from the stroke and settles into new patterns of daily life, information about the nature of the condition and the outlook for recovery begins to seem less important. Attention turns instead to finding out about the support and resources which might make living with aphasia less of a struggle.

What do people with aphasia want to know?

- *In the immediate aftermath of stroke*:
  - the cause of the stroke;
  - the range and nature of associated impairments;
  - why various impairments occur;
  - how to cope with impairments;
  - the impact of stroke on sexual function;
  - the prospect for recovery;
  - the timespan for recovery;
  - whether another stroke is likely and how to prevent this;
  - the role of various professionals;
  - what treatments and therapies are available;
  - the nature and effectiveness of treatments and therapies;
  - how long the stay in hospital is likely to be;
  - the likelihood of returning to work;
  - what support and services will be available at home;
  - what is happening with working and financial arrangements;
  - where to turn for advice and help.

- *Coming home*:
  - what services, aids and adaptations are available and how to access them;
  - whether therapies and treatments are available and how to access them;
  - the likely duration and outcome of therapies and treatments;
  - the purpose, correct useage and side-effects of medication;
  - problems which might occur, for example, fatigue and the possibility of having fits;
  - how to cope with the various impairments;
  - what the aphasic person and others can do to further recovery;
  - alternatives to working;
  - local facilities and resources which might be useful (e.g. accessible transport);
  - benefits, rights, entitlements and eligibility for support;
  - how to understand and deal with the procedures involved in making a claim;
  - where to turn for advice and help.

- *In the longer term*:
  - what services, resources and facilities are available and how to access them;

- how to cope with the long-term effects of stroke, including psychological and social issues;
- how to help other health and psychological problems within the family;
- benefits, rights, entitlements and eligibility;
- how to maintain and monitor health and how to prevent another stroke;
- where to turn for advice and help.

'The more I knew about it the better': attitudes to information

The information in the box above suggests there is a consensus about what people want to know at various stages of their aphasia. While the list does reflect the broad range of opinion, nevertheless attitudes to information can vary. For some, it is crucial. Obtaining information can bring about a feeling of reassurance, a sense of being in control and able to understand and accept what has happened.

Following her second stroke, *Jean*, who is 68, is unable to walk or use her right hand and has a mild aphasia. Her elderly husband has a visual impairment and the couple are becoming increasingly dependent on social services support. From the start, they have been given little information and have found out what they know by chance, persistence and guesswork. Initially, Jean was given no explanation of her aphasia and never had any information about how to manage that or any of the other consequences of her stroke. She thought her impairments were temporary: *'When you're taken with a stroke your life changes completely and you don't know anything. I think we should be told. — Everything seems a secret. — I thought it would only be a little while. — When you're getting well in the hospital, before you come out . . . if someone would only come and explain to you — what is available in help to the person . . . I haven't had anything to do with social workers. They should know what a person's like before they come out of hospital. — I'm the one who would rather know about things. If they tell me what's wrong and how I must fight it, I'll try. And then . . . I don't get nervous.* Jean's limited mobility and her difficulty with communication have meant that her husband has had the job of gathering information. He has found the Citizens' Advice Bureau helpful. But he has learnt most about stroke and about related issues such as disabled badges for the car (when he could drive), tax changes and special resources, through chance conversations and encounters: *'When he goes down the pub there's a man said: "Oh my wife is so-and-so." That's how you know.'*

Many people share Jean's wish to be fully informed about the outcome of their stroke and what help they can expect. But this desire cannot be assumed to be true of everyone. Some feel ambivalent about acquiring information. Reasons for this vary. It is possible to feel wary of strangers knowing about one's private business. Some feel that the process of enquiring and seeking information means they are being pushy and others that they are effectively asking for charity. Some shy away from medical information altogether, because it can confirm their worst fears about their condition, conveying knowledge which they would rather not have. It is therefore possible to have mixed feelings about seeking information and to feel anxious and upset if what is offered undermines hopes for recovery. The amount and type of information offered needs to be determined with sensitivity to the needs and feelings of the individual.

Roger still does not understand how he came to have such difficulties with communication, and wonders if he might have caught something from a beggar he encountered on a train while on holiday in Peru: *'See this chappie hobbling. Wonder this chappie diseased. Might caught it.'* Many years after his stroke occurred, he still holds out hope for a full recovery. When he sees his GP he tries to ask about this but can find the response he gets makes him feel anxious and upset: *'This brain. Better? Good? It's alright. Alright you know. It's alright now. Calm down. Calm down, you see. Help to calm down you see. But the doctors examine me, well anxie me really.'* Roger wants to know about the medication he takes and about the sudden fits of shaking he experiences, but he has trouble addressing these issues in his encounters with doctors. *'Me gone remember things.'* However, when he talks about the possibility of getting information about stroke which he can understand, perhaps in the form of a tape, he expresses his ambivalence. He also dislikes hearing about conditions which can be cured, because this forces him to acknowledge the situation in which he finds himself: *'See . . . the tape . . . hear there the tape. Me . . . depressed really. That's the problem. — Depressed, you see. It's queer, really. It's, you know, shutting down. — No. And now, funny this. Er . . . radio. And talking on the wireless see. Er . . . curing . . . curing things. Explaining things. Can't hear. Horrible. Can't. I can't hear it. You know. Irritable me. Irritable.*

'In one earhole and out the other': the problem of getting information

People who have aphasia describe four major difficulties in acquiring information. First, some are uncertain about exactly what information they need in the first place and where to locate it. Secondly, they may not always get the type and quality of information which they require. Thirdly, the ways in which information is given are often ill-suited to the needs of someone who has language difficulties. Finally, the timing of giving the information can be problematic.

Knowing what information is needed and where to locate it

Jean's experience of struggling to track down the information she needed is shared by many people. Aphasia is invisible, and perhaps this means that those whose job it is to give information may not be aware of it, or understand that it can limit a person's ability to ask questions and to enquire in person, by phone or by letter. The fact that someone with aphasia may not initiate or persist with an enquiry can be interpreted as lack of interest or need. Many aphasic people describe being left to fend for themselves in tracking information about their condition, how to cope, and the available supports and resources.

> Susan is still unsure about the cause of her stroke and how it came to cause her physical and communication impairments. She wonders whether one reason for the lack of information may be the fact that she was admitted to hospital over the Christmas period: *'They going up to the Christmas and things like that. — Why . . . what happened? I don't know. This is it. I don't know. — Could be brain clots? I don't know.'* On discharge from hospital, Susan needed information about follow-up therapies, benefits for which she might be eligible, how to prevent another stroke happening and whether or not she could claim help with the cost of new glasses. She was told nothing and didn't know that she might be eligible for services and financial support. She wonders if this might be because it was known that she had a supportive husband: *'I know really because is the my husband here so they didn't all the time. — If it is two persons alright. If it is one you mustn't, this is it. But . . . no anything . . . nothing at all. Just the hospital . . . to the hospital then back and nothing only the speech therapy, that's it. But mind I think I don't know. I didn't know it. — No services and that. — Information of health. Information on money problems. Information on . . . rights. Like glasses.'* Susan is aware of all the difficulties she would have reading information, making enquiries by phone and filling in forms, but

feels these could have been overcome. She feels that she has been left to fend for herself. Nine years after her stroke, she still doesn't know what is available or where and how to find out about it: '*Just anger. Angry this is not right. Sometimes I get angry because this is not right.*'

Susan's view that she was left to fend for herself because of the support she was receiving from her family is shared by many others. Often, relatives and friends take on the responsibility of trying to find out what has happened, what the outlook is and what help is available. Some relish the task and master the procedures involved in finding relevant information and acting upon it. But non-aphasic people may have their own difficulties tracing information. However supportive they are, relatives and friends may not find it any easier than the person who has aphasia to locate and use relevant information. Visual impairment, poor health, lack of time, limited literacy skills and lack of confidence and experience are all factors which can obstruct even the most concerned family member.

Susan's account also highlights the fact that many aphasic people are simply not aware of the existence of potential services and resources and the fact that they might be eligible for these. They do not know what they need to know:

'*The thing is, I don't know what I'm entitled to. — If you don't know where to start you never get nowhere. — I don't know. And is not just a matter of scared.*'

Vincent

Many aphasic people seem to gather bits of knowledge from a number of different sources. These can be quite random and arbitrary, ranging from chance encounters with people who have similar problems and who have had access to some service, to happening upon a poster advertising a charitable organisation which points them in the right direction:

Sources of information used by people who have aphasia

- Enquiries made by friends and family.
- The experience and advice of others passed on by word of mouth.
- Personal experience and knowledge.
- Publicity material produced by charitable organisations.
- Posters and leaflets in hospitals, post offices and libraries.
- Books.
- Service providers.

The type and quality of information given

Sometimes information can be inadequate or inaccurate. Information can be inadequate in two ways. First, those who provide information may be unaware of the very intense concerns and worries on the part of the person with aphasia and therefore these are not addressed. Secondly, only a general outline might be conveyed, possibly because it can be hard for someone with aphasia to follow up an issue, to ask detailed questions and to indicate that more is required.

Inaccurate information can be equally problematic. Some people have experience of being given information which is simply wrong. Others recall predictions about their own recovery which now seem to them to be inaccurate in either stressing a gloomy outlook or in raising hopes of a complete recovery. There are some possible explanations for this. First, people who have aphasia need information to be stated in clear, concrete and definite terms. It can be difficult to understand tentative or qualified statements although these are often necessary, for example when the long-term outcome of the stroke seems uncertain. It is possible that the people taking part in the study, who recall, for example, being told that they would definitely have full recovery, or that they definitely would never speak again, may have had to filter out all the uncertainty suggested by the person who originally gave them the information. Another possibility is that those giving information may themselves find the outlook too painful and shy away from talking about it frankly.

Following her stroke, **Sharon** remembers hearing a doctor suggest she would make a full and rapid recovery and would soon be able to walk and talk as before. She is not sure whether she heard this because it was what she wanted to hear, or because the real outlook was too upsetting for the medical staff: *'Yeah, decided alright . . . fine. Um the doctor said . . . oh yes . . . um how the doctor is well and back to normal or . . . I'm alright. Maybe. — It may have been me. I don't know . . . in my mind. Yes, alright . . . out and about maybe in two weeks' time or one weeks' time. Out and about, fit and well. — Maybe, I don't know, maybe the patient says: "Alright, a stroke, how long or . . . ?" But maybe the doctors and nurses right it's a long time. The patient says no, the doctor said may be a long time maybe um . . . the fib or liar or I . . . the doctor says to the patient: "Yes slowly getting there." — I don't know. Thinking about maybe um oh it's sad and a long time. Maybe a fib short time.'*

Many other topics which concern aphasic people are complex and may not easily be clarified or simply expressed. For example, the intricacies of the benefits system and the rapidity with which statutory changes are made and implemented means that eligibility and conditions seem constantly in a state of flux. Such changes and conditions cannot be conveyed in clear, definite terms without going into an overwhelming amount of detail.

The way in which information is given

Alf's experience highlights the particular needs which aphasic people have regarding the way in which information is given. He points out that different aphasic people will need information to be given in different ways, depending upon their needs and abilities. He likes to receive information by word of mouth, but needs a written copy to refer to so that he can retain what has been said. He needs information to be given slowly. He needs information to be repeated. He points out that those who have difficulty reading and writing may need to be contacted by someone who is willing to talk through their options at a slow pace. Alf's account illustrates commonly expressed fears and concerns.

Alf's negative experience in hospital was compounded by the fact that he was not given the information he needed to help him make sense of what was happening to him: *'I thought at first they was trying to put me in an asylum. That's what I actually thought. — I didn't know the place. I always knew it as somewhere you died. I didn't know it was a rehabilitation place. I went through the door in a wheelchair and at the same time I'm trying to fight with my left hand. You're not getting me in there. And at the same time I thought they was putting me in there to give up the struggle.'* On his return home, Alf struggled to get information about his condition and about local resources and what help he might have. He and his wife were told that he was not eligible for more financial aid: *'She was told to keep quiet because I was behind with my stamps.'* Alf tried a benefits helpline but found that the person he was talking to had never come across anyone with aphasia before. Alf ended up arguing with him about the need for him to speak slowly. He felt very nervous about contacting the Citizens' Advice Bureau for help because he knew it would place a strain on his language: *'I was going past Citizens' Advice in St Peter's Street. They had an office there. "Why am I going past them? Oh I'll just pop in and see them. Oh I can't do that." And I just couldn't make myself go to ask. — It's terrible because you cannot push yourself forward to do these things. — I have to try and copy Citizen's Advice down on a piece of paper so that I could ask them what I wanted because I never would have been able to remember what I was trying to think . . .'* Eventually, Alf did pluck up the courage to go into the Citizens' Advice Bureau, who found out he was not receiving all the financial support to which he was entitled. His daughter also pursued enquiries on his behalf. In addition, browsing through old books for sale at a local library, Alf came upon one on disability rights, and used this as a guide, both for himself and for giving advice to others. Alf is very aware of the problems encountered by people with aphasia and feels those whose job it is to give information should be trained about their needs: *'Why did I have to ask you? Why didn't you tell me? — You cannot always ask. You may not be able to speak so you're in limboland. If anybody tells you what you're entitled to, with a person who's dysphasic it goes in one earhole and out the other. It does not lodge. — If you cannot read or write, you get someone to tell you and ask them to do it slowly.'* Alf found the lack of accurate, relevant and accessible information so distressing that it made him think of suicide: *'Give up and take an overdose.'*

The timing of information

The final difficulty encountered concerns the time at which information is given. In the early stages, aphasia can place the person in a double-bind: desperately wanting to know what has happened and what is in store, yet unable to ask questions or to absorb what is said. Several people recall being offered some information at a time when they could not take it in and understand it. Even though they have therefore, technically, been provided with information, this is not their perception of what happened. People who have aphasia need information to be available at any point, in the short, middle and long term:

'I could have done with a lot more information. — I should have asked but I couldn't. I think it would have helped, but I couldn't grasp that.'

Christopher

'Two years information I think not. But two years information I stored.'

Colin

'Someone with aphasia can be plucked out': getting out of the information trap

People who have aphasia experience particular problems with getting the information they need, in the right format and at the right time. Reflecting on their experiences, many suggest ways in which the problems encountered could be resolved. The solutions cover large-scale issues relating to organisation and training within the various services as well as detailed suggestions on how the intricacies of interaction might be improved.

How can information be made accessible to people with aphasia?

- Knowing where to turn.
- Refined content and timing of information to meet individual needs.
- Regular checks on information needs.
- Supporting communication and getting the message across.

Knowing where to turn

The problem of people who have aphasia not knowing what information is needed and not knowing where to get it from could be addressed in a number of ways. A common view is that information should be pro-actively provided, that is offered without the person with aphasia having to take the initiative. This would demand proper understanding and acknowledgement of the restrictions imposed by aphasia.

'People do go without. Because they don't know who to turn to. — Everyone in our position should have a social worker come into them.'

Madge

The fact that most aphasic people seem to acquire information through chance encounters and from a haphazard combination of sources could be addressed if one person was to make contact in the early days following the stroke and maintain regular contact and support through the following years, proactively offering information relevant to the changing needs and concerns. A few people do report the reassuring effect of knowing one person with whom they maintain contact and who acts as their advocate even many years after their stroke. This would fit well with the strongly stated need for an integrated information service. It is preferable to information which is gathered in snippets from diverse agencies and sources. Aphasic people also suggest that the bureaucratic procedures of making claims could be integrated and streamlined, so that, for example, one core form could be combined with separate sections relevant to different benefits:

'Lots of forms ... long ones. Long time ago lots of forms on different things, and maybe one form with general living allowance and mobilities.'

Sharon

The content and timing of information

Aphasic people taking part in this study stress the fact that they need different types of information, on different topics as time passes and their circumstances change. The early need for medical information may give way to a need for information about services and benefits. Conversely, many years after the event, the aphasic person may want to know what a stroke is, why it occurred and what is causing the difficulties with communication. Such requirements for different types of information are idiosyncratic and unpredictable. Their diversity may obstruct a truly integrated service being offered by those from different professional backgrounds.

What seems to be required is an information service which can cross professional boundaries, which can address medical, social, welfare and other concerns, and which the aphasic person can draw upon at the appropriate time. Some people have access to local community health centres which have the potential to offer such an integrated and personalised service, but others suggest that such wide-ranging information needs should be addressed by the voluntary and charitable organisations. The Stroke Association is developing a network of stroke information centres across the UK in an attempt to address this need. However, at the time of interview of the people who took part in the study none was aware of or had made use of this service. Whichever agency provides an information service, a commonly held view is that it should be proactive in addressing the individual needs of the aphasic person over time. Personnel should have special training in order to enable and support the best possible communication.

Regular checks on information needs

Many aphasic people point out that they may need to be offered the same information several times over the period following their stroke. For example, Annie has benefited from listening several times over to the standard explanation of aphasia which the speech and language therapist gives to new people joining the therapy group. She appreciates the thoughtfulness with which such information sessions are integrated into the sessions. Others point out that information cannot simply be repeated without taking account of what the aphasic person's information needs are. They suggest the need for a systematic way of registering these and how they are changing over time, perhaps in the form of questionnaires or interviews which could be administered at regular intervals. Again, this would demand the consistent involvement of personnel who are trained in supporting communication.

Getting the message across

Aphasic people suggest many different ways in which their access to information could be improved, depending on their particular needs and abilities. The diverse nature of aphasia means that each person has individual requirements which need to be checked out by those providing information. Leaving a written record of a conversation may be helpful to one aphasic person and of little use to another. Similarly, one person may be helped if written information is read aloud, another may be distracted by too much going on at once, and so on. The ideas suggested in the box below should not, therefore, be taken as universally applicable to interaction with all people who have aphasia.

Supporting communication and getting the message across

- Take a calm, friendly, respectful and encouraging approach.
- Try not to rush the aphasic person, however busy you are.
- Make sure the aphasic person understands the purpose of the conversation.
- Ask the aphasic person to let you know what is and is not helpful.
- Talk directly to the person who has aphasia, maintaining eye contact and watching body language.
- Talk slowly.
- Regularly check that the aphasic person is understanding what is being said and the topic.
- Use straightforward language and avoid jargon.
- Repeat information as required.
- Using an interpreter if necessary, make sure written and spoken information is provided in the appropriate language.
- Note down key points covered in the conversation and leave this as a record.
- Highlight or underline key points in leaflets.
- Back up explanations and questions with diagrams and drawings if necessary. Always have paper and pencil to hand and make sure you write clearly.
- Use analogies (for example, likening the bloodflow in the brain to a road network which gets blocked at one point, forcing traffic to move to another route).
- Make a tape recording of the conversation which the person can refer to later.
- Ask questions in a form which can be understood, using drawing, writing and keywords if necessary.
- Work through leaflets and forms at the aphasic person's pace.
- Make sure all written information is clearly laid out and simply expressed in key points.
- Encourage the aphasic person to use any means of communication, including drawing, writing and pointing to key words or pictures.

These basic points offer some ground rules for making information more accessible to people with aphasia in a one-to-one exchange. However, much written information which is currently available does not meet the need for simplicity and clarity of expression. While some aphasic people are aware of the potential of video-based and computerised information systems which could cover different topics at different levels of complexity and be used interactively, it is clear that the provision of written information will not be developed in an appropriate way unless a strong case is made for removing the textual obstacles faced by aphasic people. Those who are best qualified to do this are restricted by the nature of their impairment.

In addition, aphasic people are aware that their requirements concerning the form, nature and content of information are likely to be costly. Meeting such needs would involve long-term commitment, training for personnel and the provision of consistent, individualised support. Some point out that making information accessible may not be high on the agenda:

'The thing is, it's all put into so many words precisely to stop people claiming.'
Christopher

The experience of trying to access information can cause as much anger, frustration and distress to aphasic people as their physical and linguistic impairments. It is possible to feel more disabled by the lack of relevant and understandable information, than by loss of movement or difficulty locating a word.

The struggle to get information continues to prove very stressful for **Ravi**, who had a heart attack prior to his stroke. Years after the event, he is still uncertain about what happened to him, what the outlook is, the precise purpose of his medication and whether an operation to clear his blocked arteries contributed to his stroke: *'I don't know exactly what has happened.'* A number of factors contribute to his difficulties. His consultant, whom he has not seen for two years, and his GP disagree about the correct dosage for his medication, so he receives contradictory instructions which he finds confusing. He finds it an ordeal to negotiate an appointment with the receptionist at the doctor's surgery: *'If I phone them this morning that I want to see the doctor . . . urgent . . . now . . . "How can you valify that?" '* When he does manage to get an appointment, his GP gives him little time to talk. This makes Ravi upset, angry and less able to communicate: *'He's not even taking a time for me. — Rush, rush, rush. — I have been frustrated and inside me I feel as if what do I do now? — It takes me two or three days to get* *settled again.'* Ravi's problems with communication affect his ability to find out about services and resources. He shies away from using the phone to enquire about a bus pass, because he cannot explain his aphasia to the person on the other end of the line. He is over-whelmed by the complexity and length of information and forms relating to benefits and has to rely on his wife, who has limited literacy in English: *'My wife is not that much educated, you know. When you say education this means the complications of all the forms and things like that. So you have someone like my son or my daughter.'* For Ravi, the seemingly constant changes in the benefits system remind him of his experiences under Amin's regime, which forced him to flee Uganda: *'Everything is at loggerheads against it is that . . . loggerhead everywhere. — Sometimes we need to feel as if it was . . . I come from Uganda, you know, so that time, when that person was there. — That that thing what was happening there, it is happening today. Because everything . . . switch on the telly there is a new rule, something that change. You are not going to get this benefit. Every second was changing. — To get a pound from the benefit, you are to fill in such a form, so many forms so that you feel that it's better not to bother.'*

7

'Doing the inside work':
the meaning of aphasia

Aphasia is difficult to understand, both for those who have it and for those who do not. It cannot be seen or felt, it can take different forms, it is unpredictable, and it affects a number of processes which are rarely thought about in any conscious way, such as putting words in the right order and understanding what others say. Yet it has a major impact on every aspect of life and, as such, it has to be dealt with. People who have aphasia endeavour to understand it, explain it and, ultimately, cope with it. This chapter will explore the ways in which aphasic people talk and think about their language impairment. It will look at the ways in which they explain aphasia, both to themselves and others, and the things they do to make living with aphasia easier.

'As I talked, the words was tumbling': descriptions of aphasia

Physicians and therapists may seek to explain particular aspects of aphasia to their patients. They may try to convey information about the cause and nature of the impairment, and are concerned with identifying particular signs and 'symptoms' which have clinical significance. However, it seems that people who have aphasia do not always see these in the same way as the professionals. Indeed, aspects of aphasia which individuals consider important and relevant may not be the same as those which concern clinicians. In giving their account of aphasia, people can focus on a number of different aspects.

What is aphasia? Aspects described by aphasic people

- The onset of aphasia.
- The causes and physical nature of aphasia.
- Emotional responses to aphasia.
- What aphasia feels like.
- Language breakdown.

Some aspects of aphasia, such as its onset and the range and intensity of emotions which it can trigger, are often described in such full and vivid detail that they become relatively easy for someone who does not have aphasia to appreciate. Other aspects tend to be described in a more faltering and hesitant way, suggesting that these are perhaps more difficult to understand and to express.

Emotional responses to aphasia

People who have aphasia are able to talk in a detailed way about its emotional impact, and how this has changed from the time of onset to the present day. Becoming aware, in the beginning, that communication is a struggle, that people are not understanding what is said, that the written word does not make sense anymore, is a frightening and bewildering experience. Initially, aphasia seems to bring about a tumult of conflicting emotions, including amusement, fury and despair, which are hard to get under control and difficult to forget. Thinking and talking about the shock of the first days can bring back intense and distressing memories.

The consequences of aphasia slowly unfold. Years after the onset of the impairment, as they take stock of its impact, people still describe the sense of being subject to strong emotions.

For **Stephen**, the onset of aphasia came as a major blow. It meant he had to leave the work he loved. He lost contact with friends and colleagues and became increasingly reliant on his wife and family for company. Eight years after his stroke, Stephen still struggles with feelings of fear and panic when he goes out: *'Blooming scared — of just everything.'* Touching his chest, to show how his heart pounds when he meets people, he says: *'I mean is er . . . not pur . . . purgatory but is em . . . like bom, bom, bom, bom, bom.'* For Stephen, company is essential but difficult to seek out because of his aphasia and because this goes against his natural reserve. He has now made contact with a group of aphasic people, who offer support and social contact but still feels that his relationships with others lack depth, because of aphasia: *'All relationship is missing . . . round the corner.'* Left alone, he finds himself prey to feelings of depression and worthlessness, which perhaps other people do not see: *'I love work. I love work and it's no good. — Eight years ago is on the telephone chat chat chat all day for me. And now is finished. — It's a blank. — My speech is just tongue-tied. Unbelievable is so awful. — Once in a blue moon is like scream. — Sitting indoors is a bit bore . . . bored, so I want to go out. To me is always smiling and happy but inside's like . . . like maybe indoors, cup of tea and like because I can't think, it strikes me bad just thinking. Indoors, just me myself, sit down and's nothing.'*

As time passes, the intense emotions stirred by the experience of aphasia slowly start to fall into more clearly defined patterns. The most commonly described feelings are those of frustration, anger and embarrassment. These can be triggered by a number of different situations, for example, struggling to ask for a busfare, telling a joke, or a chance encounter with neighbours while out shopping. It is possible to deal with these emotions in a number of ways. Some aphasic people become increasingly isolated, giving up their attempts at interaction with the outside world. Some restrict their social world, having contact only with members of the family and small groups of friends whom they know will understand. Others channel their strong feelings into assertive or sometimes antagonistic behaviour towards others. Different ways of handling the emotions lead to several possible outcomes including depression, a sense of increasing confidence as contacts are maintained and developed, and resignation to the way things are. Individuals pursue their own pathways through the complex layers of emotions, responses and strategies to reach these different outcomes. In addition, if an aphasic person becomes depressed early on (which can happen as one of the biochemical consequences of damage to the brain), then this will affect the way in which the person deals with aphasia, and can reduce the number of strategies available.

While it may be true that emotional responses to aphasia can become more stable and predictable as time passes, this should not mask the swings of feeling which can still occur years after the stroke, nor the intensity of the distress which can be experienced. The accounts given in this study show that, for some people, the difficulties associated with loss of communication are so severe they can lead to thoughts of suicide.

The causes and physical nature of aphasia

Some people think about and describe their aphasia in terms of its physical causes and manifestations, perhaps because these aspects seem more concrete and easier to grasp. Most people locate the source of the problem within the brain, but a small number explain it almost as a form of laryngitis or as a form of muscular weakness. Those who do talk about their impairment in terms of brain function can understandably find themselves struggling with the detail of this. They usually confine themselves to quite general statements and leave it at that. However, some people take the explanation further, conveying the sense that the brain seems to have lost control over the parts of the body used for speaking or writing.

Aphasia explained in physical terms

- As a form of laryngitis or muscular weakness:
  'I realise it's in my throat.'

    Harold

    'It's taken my voice.'

    Jean

    Asked what aphasia is, **Jack** touches the right side of his face.

- As a result of something which has happened to the brain:
  'Something to do with the brain.'

    Janet

    'It's a physical problem relating to the mind.'

    Edward

    'A blood clot went over the brain and that's partly what causes the speech.'

    Fred

- As a disconnection between the brain and the means of speaking and writing:
  'My brain is just buzzing about and me lips is a different kettle of fish.'

    Stephen

    'I cannot get the brain and the hand to work together.'

    Geoffrey

    'The brain is thinking. He cannot get the words out, but he's thinking.'

    Alf

What aphasia feels like

Using images which, in their different ways, evoke feelings of emptiness and isolation, some people try to convey a sense of what the experience of aphasia is like.

Images used to describe what aphasia feels like

*'That has all gone and I can't bring it out. It's just as if there's an empty space.
— Like opening doors and there's nothing in there. But that is the only way
I could describe it.
It was just as if my brain was a cake and a piece of it was cut out.'*

Betty

'My brains had gone off on holiday.'

Mike

'I got blocked.'

Susan

'A rose tightly shut and a bit wilting.'

Rose

*'As far as I was concerned, I was talking and I was explaining things. But the
people are statues looking blank. It's a funny feeling that, when you're talking ... I don't know what the sound is like but the words and all that
sounded in the head ... I got the impression, like the first weeks, that I had a
hole in my head and I could see the words tumbling down there. It's very
queer.'*

Les

Such images succeed in conveying some of the disturbing sensations
brought about by aphasia. They stand in marked contrast to the brief
descriptions of the physical aspects of aphasia, and those which address
the fact that it concerns the breakdown of language.

Aphasia as a breakdown of language

Most people seem to struggle when describing the problems with language which they experience. Some focus on separate functions or
components of language, which are picked out because they are not
working properly. Other people try to define what is happening to their
language by detailing the functions which are not affected. These descriptions are frequently brief and matter-of-fact. This stands in contrast to the
rich language and imagery which many people use to convey the emotions and sensations associated with their aphasia.

Descriptions of aphasia as a breakdown of language

- Isolated components of language which are not working:

  'I can't remember people's names.'

  Betty

  'I cannot read. I cannot write. I cannot spell.'

  Mike

  'I have the feelings that I can't talk properly.'

  Gladys

  'I know the right word, but the wrong word comes out.'

  Rose

  'I can't say a lot of the long, complicated words.'

  Geoffrey

- Defining aphasia by what it is not:

  'In my mind it's alright. Speaking out is naff.'

  Sharon

  'No problem with the mental attitude.'

  Douglas

Using the words 'language' and 'aphasia'

What is striking about all the different accounts of aphasia given by aphasic people is that two words rarely occur. With very few exceptions, people do not talk about 'language' and they do not talk about 'aphasia'. Thinking about language does not seem to come naturally. During an ordinary conversation, those taking part pay attention to what is said, to the message that is being transmitted, and to the way in which it is said. But it is rare to think consciously about the system that makes the conversation possible and to consider all the separate components and processes involved: selecting which aspect of an event to convey; finding the right words to do this; arranging them in the correct order; producing speech sounds and at the same time monitoring and processing what is being said. Indeed, few people would break language down into such component parts. These only attract conscious attention when a language is being learnt or when something goes wrong, when a word is pronounced in a curious way, the structure of a sentence sounds odd, when the person seems to be missing the point or struggling to find a word.

By making things go wrong, aphasia forces people to focus on the components, the nuts and bolts of language. They are confronted with a number of things they can no longer do: finding words; making grammatical sentences; spelling; reading; talking. Separate functions attract attention, but are not linked together and not understood as part of the breakdown of a general system — which is precisely what the term 'aphasia' refers to. Many aphasic people have heard the term but freely admit they have no idea what it is. Others are aware that they have aphasia, and that it is important, but struggle to define it.

Some definitions of aphasia

'It's a person who does not know his left from his right, who's had an operation or a stroke and it's called aphasic'.

Alf

'Aphasia is no speech or conversation.'

Robert

'Aphasia? You mean stroke?'

Tom

'Aphasia is something weird.'

Lionel

'Obviously, I have got a problem with . . . phasi.'

Edward

'All I know is that I don't know what aphasia is.'

Philip

This issue is complicated by a number of other factors. 'Aphasia' is an unusual sounding word, which can be difficult to say. The thought of using it and trying to explain it to others can be alarming. The fact that the words 'aphasia' and 'dysphasia' are used interchangeably contributes to the sense of confusion surrounding the term. But, most obviously, the very people who are struggling to take on a new concept and learn the term for it, find that the very nature of their impairment makes this difficult to do.

Reasons why the term 'aphasia' is rarely used

- It refers to the concept of a general language system, which may be unfamiliar.
- Componential nature of aphasia leads to focus on separate functions: *'It's being able to speak and pronounce and I forget the others.'*
- Difficult word, both to say and to explain: *'All the time: "Asphasia? What is that?"'*
- 'Aphasia' and 'dysphasia' used interchangeably, adding to confusion: *'I think dysphasia is a term, but aphasia is not.'*
- Aphasia is not easily identifiable and can differ from person to person.
- Aphasia makes it difficult to take on and use new vocabulary: *'It takes me a lot of time to get used to any new words.'*

'I get Ken to do it': practical strategies used by people with aphasia

Although the concept of aphasia may be difficult to take on and to express, it is nevertheless possible to develop many different ways and practical strategies which make living with aphasia easier. People with aphasia operate three main kinds of practical strategies which make living with aphasia easier: using aids and appliances (such as spellcheckers and answerphones); enlisting the help of other people (for example, asking someone to talk with the bank manager on their behalf); and changing aspects of their own communication (for example, moving away from noisy environments, giving extra time to reading, jotting down a list of points to be covered before making a phone call). Not all strategies will be useful for everyone. Individuals set up the systems which work best for them.

Such strategies are only helpful in supporting very basic aspects of communication — the giving and receiving of information. They do not help the aphasic person to get across or receive more complex ideas, or to enjoy the more subtle aspects of language, for example joking and punning with friends. Other strategies which are helpful in allowing aphasic people more access to communication may be difficult to identify. This is because they involve making changes in the way people talk. Someone who has aphasia might only have access to a conversation if certain requirements are met. Thus, a discussion might need to be conducted more slowly, and perhaps punctuated with frequent breaks. The points covered and the conclusions reached may need to be summarised at regular intervals and checked with the aphasic person. The fact that different aphasic people may have different requirements adds to the difficulty of doing this in an appropriate way. It also reinforces the need for non-aphasic people to 'check out' with aphasic speakers what helps and what does not help. No one rule applies to all. If the aphasic person is consulted and frequent checks are made, then it is less likely the non-aphasic person will behave in a patronising or otherwise inappropriate way.

As well as developing practical strategies for making communication easier, people who have aphasia find ways of relieving the sadness, stress, bitterness and other unpleasant emotions which they might feel. In order to achieve this, individuals draw on ways of thinking which they may have used for years before the onset of aphasia, when dealing with sad or troublesome feelings. Methods used by one person may not suit another.

Feeling better: ways of relieving sad or troublesome thoughts and emotions

- Compare self with others: *'Some of em's worse than what I am.'*
- Share experiences with others: *'We're all in the same boat.'*
- Humour: *'We've had a lot of laughs . . . laughing . . . laughter over it.'*
- Adopt an attitude of resignation: *'I've become accustomed to what I am.'*
- Spirituality, prayer and meditation: *'Speak and silence and prayer — I've found something different speak and understand.'*
- Take stock of progress to date: *'I gone on one hundred per cent.'*
- Talk to friends: *'When I talk to them I get it all out . . . all my steam.'*
- Count one's blessings: *'I'm very lucky to be alive anywhere.'*

What does 'coping with aphasia' mean?

The practical ways in which aphasic people make life easier represent one aspect of coping with the impairment. But learning to cope with a suddenly acquired, long-term condition such as aphasia is not just a simple matter of developing strategies or finding ways of feeling better. It is an essential and complex process, which is not fully understood, whereby the person strives to make sense of the new situation in personal terms. In this more general sense, coping means trying to account for what has happened and what will happen. It is a process in which the person with aphasia reaches an understanding of how life was before, how and why it has changed, what has helped or limited recovery, and how life might be in the future.

'Coping' generally has positive overtones, but this can be deceptive. It is not necessarily a matter of 'looking on the bright side' or finding the positive aspects of the new situation. Of course, some people can cope with aphasia by making a new life for themselves, but others may cope in very different ways – for example, by listing and regretting their losses, by becoming angry at the therapy or treatment they have received, or by trying to dismantle the obstacles they face. So different people will cope in different ways, giving different accounts of their aphasia. An essential feature of coping is that it involves the aphasic person actively making an account of what has happened which makes sense to them. It is therefore constructive, even though it might not be positive.

At the time of her stroke, which happened when she was 26, **Emma** was married and had a demanding job working in insurance. Her life changed completely. She underwent years of intensive private treatment and rigorous rehabilitation, backed up by family and friends. This has only recently stopped. Her marriage broke up, she was no longer able to work and now lives close to her parents. Having lost contact with many of her own friends, Emma has recently had to start building up a new social circle, and draws upon the support of her parents' friends and neighbours. Recently, she has started to see some old school friends who have also been through the trauma of divorce. Eight years after her stroke, Emma is still taking stock of the major changes in her situation, prospects, and in attributes which she had felt to be an intrinsic part of her character: *'I'd like to be able to work again but I won't do that. My professor doesn't think I'll able to earn a wage . . . I was ever so fast in my job and in speaking as well . . . I'm not a fast-speaking person, unlike before.'* Perhaps because of the intensity of the physical and language rehabilitation she experienced, Emma has tended to see both her body and her language as machines which have broken down. Fixing them has been the job of professionals and experts. She does not see herself as having taken an active part in this process. Instead, she has been worked upon and dealt with by others: *'My father sorted it out because at the time I couldn't understand and I was in a dreadful situation . . . My mum and dad pulled me through . . . You worked towards the family keeping on at me and on at me. People worked on me . . . they came and did my exercises on Saturday.'* Now the regime of therapies has come to an end, Emma is starting to face the idea that the prospects for further improvement are slim, but it is hard to let go of the spirit of hopefulness which accompanies treatment: *'I go from day to day thinking it'll be improved . . . I'd like to be more positive about things. I got to go on living. I get a little bit depressed sometimes, but I not got to think about that.'* Emma's account suggests that she continues to regret her losses and to hope for an improvement through rehabilitation. She is only now starting to acknowledge that her difficulties with communication might be here to stay and is naturally, upset by this. She does not have a clear idea of what aphasia is. Because of the vitality of her previous life, the shock of so many major changes and the gruelling experience of rehabilitation, she is only now starting to think ahead, and to contemplate her future life. This is a lonely and difficult process, partly because she is not sure what skills, attributes and abilities she has. Her various therapies did not address these matters and she has been left to work things out for herself. She has never met anyone else who has aphasia and therefore has no way of defining what has happened to her in relation to the experiences of others.

Emma's account suggests how complex and long drawn out the process of coping can be. One way of breaking down this complex process is to construct a model of what seems to be happening, based upon people's accounts. The model in Figure 7.1 shows how the process of coping is continuous and on-going, and how it seems to involve the interaction of a number of different stages and components:

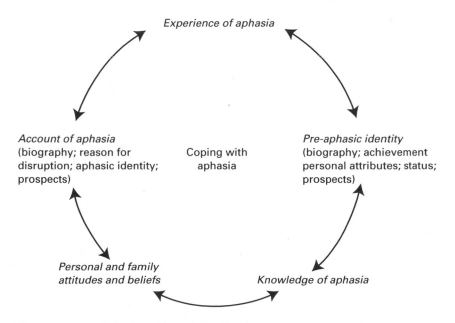

Figure 7.1 Model of coping with aphasia

The impact of aphasia upon identity

Before they become aphasic, people are absorbed in finding a way through their achievements, failures, hopes and ambitions. They are not only busy getting on with the present, but also with looking back and looking forward as they take stock and make plans. This continuous, on-going process makes up their biography, their personal story. The experience of aphasia suddenly interrupts the biography of the person who develops it. It is associated with changes in many aspects of life: work; education; relationships; domestic organisation; and even personal attributes such as wit or ease of conversation, which might have seemed to be fundamental and unalterable characteristics. All these features make up a person's identity, or sense of self. They also contribute to the person's sense of status, or location of self in relation to others. When they are altered by aphasia, the person's sense of identity and status become fragile and vulnerable. People who develop aphasia temporarily lose their bearings. Their past becomes untenable and their future becomes uncertain.

Drawing on knowledge of aphasia, attitudes and beliefs

The aphasic person starts to cope with the changes by trying to find out what has happened, what the problem is and what the prospects are. Whatever knowledge is gleaned mixes in with personal and family attitudes and beliefs regarding illness and recovery. For example, the person may believe that some stressful event may have caused the stroke, that it was caught from someone else, or that it was punishment for reckless living. A number of factors might be believed to affect recovery: personal determination and persistent hard work; access to enough therapy, or the right kind of therapy; the passing of time or the ministrations of healers. Differing beliefs about the cause, nature or appropriate treatment for aphasia can be a cause of conflict between family members. Sometimes, too, the aphasic person's beliefs may clash with those of medical or therapeutic professionals. For example, the widely held belief that significant recovery can continue for years after the onset of aphasia is often met with a sceptical response from therapists and medical personnel.

Constructing an account of aphasia

Drawing on experience, knowledge and belief, the person who has aphasia starts to construct an account of what has happened. This incorporates the pre-stroke biography or personal history, the nature of and reasons for changes which have occurred, the ways in which recovery has been helped or hindered. In line with their accounts of what has happened, some people start to construct new identities for themselves. These can take many forms.

Some people feel themselves to be figures engaged in a heroic battle against their condition, which they defeat by drawing upon personal qualities such as persistence, determination and stoicism. Some present themselves, and others in the same situation, as central players in a tragedy in which they have lost everything, including all their former abilities and attributes. Some find a new identity and status in helping others. They become problem-fixers or advisers. Some become experts in recording their condition, using professional terms to detail the symptoms and changes they observe. Some seek to inspire others by demonstrating the miraculous changes they have undergone in the course of recovery. Some feel themselves to be victims of poor or inadequate services, and become concerned with attaching blame to some person or situation. Some see themselves as a broken-down machine, which needs to be fixed by an expert. Some contemplate the barriers with which they are faced and become activists, tackling the stigma and oppression which help to make the impairment of aphasia into a disability.

Examples of different identities used in dealing with aphasia

- Dogged fighter: '*Is mind over matter. I've . . . I've persevere. Long, hard struggle.*'
- Recovered against the odds: '*They won't believe I had a massive stroke. I tell them I couldn't speak. They think I'm wonderful.*'
- Helper and adviser: '*I say "Keep persevering and carry on and God be with you and help you." '*
- Campaigner: '*Because they can't talk doesn't mean they're any less intel-ligent or any less capable. — People should be educated about aphasia.*'
- Tragic figure: '*Some people realise and say: "Oh, you've had a terrible life" and it's true. It's true.*'
- Machine which needs fixing: '*The brain. Doing something? Doing something?*'

Two features add to the complexity of this process. First, people do not use just one identity and one account of aphasia. Most people mix and match according to different situations, and the feelings and beliefs of those around them. Inevitably, the personal account of aphasia will be influenced by the beliefs of those who are closest to the aphasic person. Sometimes families agree on the identity of the aphasic person, but there can be conflicts. No one account is better or more desirable than another, but some will fit more snugly with the views of others, including pro-fessional or voluntary care-givers. Thus, it may be easier for a therapist, consultant or volunteer to work with someone who takes the identity of a dogged fighter, than with someone who is an angry victim.

Secondly, the process of coping is continuous, on-going and changes over time. New experiences of living with aphasia are constantly being fed into the account. The aphasic person continually looks for evidence, for signs which will back up the theories under construction. Progressing through the events of acute illness, treatment and recovery, the aphasic person will find a number of different accounts and identities useful. Coping, in this sense, is a messy and untidy business. There are no neat stages through which the aphasic person progresses in an orderly and predictable manner.

Kiran's stroke and resulting aphasia led to changes in most aspects of his life. It was *'a God-damn explosive thing to happen.'* He was no longer able to continue his work, his first marriage broke up and some close friends lost contact with him. He also found that his aphasia took away the speed of wit and the way with words which had been so much part of him, a loss which is much more significant to him than the physical changes he has also had to deal with. The loss of humour robbed him of one of the main ways he had of dealing with life events. Taking stock of all this, he says: *'Basically, I feel powerlessness. That is the hardest thing. And my language is all a part of the world. Even now, I get fed up with writing with my left hand . . . I'm annoyed with myself. I feel frustrated with myself for not spelling words correctly. My grammar is affected. I can only operate in my writing in simple sentences . . . My whole being is changed. I was always a performer and now I can't perform . . . I'm garrulous. I like to tell funny stories and it is hard for me to adapt.'* For Kiran, such fundamental changes in his identity are painful. Different aspects of his character have started to take precedence. He is working to reconcile the past and the present: *'I'm depressed but this depression is necessary for me to do the inside work . . . I mean working psychologically . . . I'm healing myself. I've come to respect myself much more than I previously had . . . You have to suffer to gain anything.'* Kiran is striving to acknowledge his old self, let it go, and to get to know the skills and attributes he now has: *'I always compare myself . . . when I'm in front of the mirror I see Kiran Mark One. But I'm Kiran Mark Two. That is the hardest part . . . I have changed. I want to become the Kiran Mark Two . . . I'm finding it hard to take the new Kiran along as I am now.'* Kiran's new self has many attributes. *'I am a good listener now, because I have to be . . . I will not apologise for my speech. I'm fed up of saying I'm sorry. I'm a fighter and being a victim doesn't fit easy to my character . . . I've come to be responsible for myself.'* While he has hopes that his recovery will continue, at this stage Kiran faces many challenges. He has to find ways in which the barriers which block his return to meaningful work can be removed, to develop his potential, build his confidence in the fact that he is valued by his friends and become able to ask for assistance, something that still bothers him: '*I feel ashamed to ask for help.*' Kiran has established contact with others who have aphasia. He both offers support and draws on the experience and strength of others. He wishes to be supported by, and to offer support to, those around him: '*I want to change myself in a society that has responsibility for me, and I have a responsibility to it.*'

Kiran's account shows how he is building his new identity on the basis of acknowledging his current abilities and attributes, together with the limitations and requirements imposed by aphasia. Moving out from his personal struggle, he is contemplating the barriers and obstacles which impede his own progress and that of others. He no longer needs to define himself by his previous skills and achievements. He is pushing his boat out.

Those who forge such a new identity seek to reconcile their former and their new selves, and to move on from the changes. Some also re-establish a collective identity, the sense of being part of communities and groups, by drawing on and providing support for others who have aphasia. Such people tend to adopt a more activist view than those who see their role as providing help or inspiration. Although hoping for further recovery and requiring specific forms of support, they start to take responsibility for living with aphasia. This is a complex, delicate and often protracted process. Kiran's term 'the inside work' hints at the effort required.

'*All I know is that I don't know what aphasia is*': the role of language in coping

It is difficult to know to what degree aphasia interferes with people's ability to cope with it in the more general terms of constructing an account which makes sense. The evidence from this study suggests that people with aphasia are as able as anyone to build their own accounts and identities. It is possible even for those who have more severe impairments to convey some aspects of their account, as Jack demonstrated when he communicated the fact that he is angry at the limited amount of therapy he received.

Despite the nature of their impairment, some people are able to give a good idea of what their version of the story is by using images, and selecting particular vocabulary and grammatical structures. Thus Roger, who has quite a marked aphasia, effectively conveys his sense of having been rendered passive and inert by using short phrases in which the same grammatical form is repeated. Using this means, he shows how he sees himself, in some ways, as the object or recipient of the attentions and activities of others:

'Taught me. — Organised me. — Watching me, guarding me. Assist me. Assist me. Lift me. — Safe me, supporting me.'

However, it is likely that aphasia affects some components of the process of coping. For example, it may limit knowledge and understanding of what aphasia is, making it hard for a person to understand the explanations and the prospects, and to add these into the formula. Severe language impairment may make it very much more difficult for the person to revisit the old self and to work on the construction of the new, because this process is often conducted through language, through talk and discussion. For those with marked impairment, this process of reconstruction may have to go on under the surface of language. Certainly, difficulties with communication will make it hard for people with aphasia to share their interpretations, to understand other people's accounts, to be listened to by those closest to them and those whose job it is to support them. Being able to talk about aphasia may help a person to capture and give shape and detail to their ideas, understanding and beliefs. The impairment damages this facility. It seems that language, while not essential for coping, may nevertheless enrich and diversify the process, and offer people more choice and scope in how they choose to live with aphasia.

8

'They cannot see it so how will they know?': aphasia and disability

Although they talk in detail about the experience of living with aphasia and the frustrations it brings, few people regard their loss of language as a disability. The reasons for this are complex, but have their source in the ambiguous nature of aphasia and the tangle of issues which surrounds the concept of disability. This chapter will draw on the accounts of aphasic people in attempting to unravel different beliefs about disability in general and attitudes to others who have aphasia. It will explore whether, and to what extent people who have aphasia are disabled.

'To me, that is someone who has lost the use of their arms and legs': aphasia and personal views of disability

Like other people, those with aphasia have different and individual understandings of disability. These draw on long-established personal attitudes and beliefs and on past and perhaps more recent experiences of meeting disabled people in hospitals, rehabilitation settings and day centres. Many people associate the idea of disability with physical and sensory impairments, especially those which can be seen, and which are clearly marked out by equipment such as a wheelchair or a white stick. In addition, the term 'disabled' is often used with reference to a person's eligibility for support, in the form of concessions and benefits. The accounts given in this study suggest that disability is seen as something which is easily identifiable, long-lasting and unlikely to get better: a definite, stable and long-term state. For many, 'the disabled' are clearly marked out by their visible impairments.

Aphasia does not fit comfortably with such perceptions of disability for a number of reasons. First, it cannot be seen:

'You can see a person in a wheelchair . . . he or she got no legs. Then you say: "Oh yes. That person is disabled." But you cannot see that I am aphasic. They cannot see it, so how will they know? Have I got to have a noticeboard up and say: "I am aphasic" '?

Alf

Secondly, aphasia is not always regarded as being a stable and consistent state. Many people comment that their own aphasia can be unpredictable, depending on the situation and levels of stress and fatigue. It can be a severe problem one day and a relatively minor hindrance the next. Aphasia also varies from person to person. It can take many different forms and may vary in severity, making it difficult to recognise in others. In addition, it is associated with acute and dramatic illness, with the result that many people feel initially that their aphasia is a temporary state, from which they will continue to recover. Perhaps most significantly, aphasia is difficult to understand and to identify, for reasons which were explored in the last chapter. All these features make aphasia ambiguous and difficult to grasp, characteristics which aphasic people may not associate with disability. They also make it, in some ways, similar to some other 'hidden' impairments, such as epilepsy or deafness.

Reasons why aphasia does not fit easily with perceptions of disability

- It is not visible: *'To look at me, it doesn't look as if you've had a stroke.'*
- It can be unpredictable: *'Up and down you know. Like Thursday is fine and maybe like Thursday week is bad. Like a yo-yo.'*
- It varies from person to person: *'Everybody's different. My friends . . . she can talk better, so much better.'*
- It can be difficult to recognise aphasia in others: *'I wasn't the same category.'*
- It is not generally understood: *'We asked them all what aphasia meant and nobody knew.'*
- It is associated with illness and recovery: *'It's an illness. Means that my brain is damaged slightly. It takes at least five years to recover ninety per cent. Recovery can go on for a long time more.'*

'I feel very sorry for them': aphasia and joining with others

Aphasia is difficult to identify and understand in personal terms. But it can also be difficult to identify and understand in others. Many aphasic people do not associate their own struggles with those of other aphasic people. They do not see themselves as part of a group of people who face common issues and who have common concerns. There are a number of possible reasons for this.

Why is it difficult for people who have aphasia to identify with others?

- Aphasic people may not be able to find others, to discuss and compare situations, and to organise action as a group.
- Aphasia is ambiguous and varies from person to person. This makes it hard to recognise others in the same situation.
- The context in which they meet can affect how aphasic people see each other.
- Aphasic people may not always wish to associate themselves with others and to work together on an equal footing.

Finding and recognising others who have aphasia

The nature of aphasia makes it difficult to find others in a similar situation. The communication impairment itself may mean that aphasic people cannot ask for or understand information about possible contact with others and make or understand arrangements. In addition, because it is ambiguous and variable, aphasia may not always be identified. Unlike deaf people who may be able to communicate using an established sign language, those who have aphasia have no common 'aphasic language' which everyone can use and understand. Cut off by the lack of communication, people who have aphasia are not always able to compare notes with others, and indeed may struggle to understand them. Without common ground, many people feel isolated and resort to looking inwards to find explanations and solutions to the problems they face.

The effect of context on meeting with others

Aphasic people who are able to meet others do so in a variety of settings. They encounter others in hospital wards, rehabilitation units, day centres, stroke clubs and social groups organised and run by charities and voluntary organisations and self-help groups. However, the difficulty with communication means that they may have to rely on these pre-established forms of contact which have been set up by others. The different contexts can affect the ethos of encounters with others. In the hospital ward, the emphasis naturally falls on recovery from illness and treatment. Many aphasic people point out that meeting others in hospital helped them to understand their own situation. Comparison with others enabled them to work out how serious it was. This could be uplifting or depressing, but was often the only form of information which they could take in at the time. Some people joined with others at this very early stage, in joking, keeping each other's spirits up and coping with the rigours of treatment.

Meeting others in a rehabilitation setting, the emphasis continues to fall on treatment and making progress. In this environment, while a feeling of solidarity may develop, the progress of the individual is still paramount. Comparison with others enables people with aphasia to understand their own progress and their own limitations. Later, meeting up in stroke clubs, day centres and in groups which focus on language games and activities, many aphasic people value the opportunity to interact and relax with others. The caring ethos of the clubs, which are often run by volunteers in association with professionals, reduces isolation and brings a sense of being supported. While these are valuable outcomes, such an atmosphere does not necessarily promote a sense of actively joining together. Lack of language means that aphasic people are often placed in situations in which they are passive recipients of care. Such environments can reinforce the impression that people are there, not to help themselves, but to be helped and to be 'done to':

'The people that do all that sit round the tables. They persons who take the tables — volunteers, the volunteers. — Their job is to get them to talk.'

Martha

Those who join the self-help groups which are springing up all over the United Kingdom describe a different ethos.

Alf has joined with others in a self-help group. For him, this kind of contact with others is important and he looks on it as a starting point for discussion, campaigning and action: *'This is now what you call self-help. Marvellous, marvellous. — I do talk more than I should do only because I'm trying to encourage other people to talk, question, disagree. — You know there's help if you want it. Without these people you wouldn't be strong enough to help each other through the government.'* Alf's experience of aphasia makes him increasingly aware of others who are vulnerable. On a recent hospital stay, he identified the fact that a Panjabi-speaking family sitting around the bed of his neighbour in the ward were completely bewildered by aphasia, and appeared not to have been given any information they could understand: *'I went into the waiting room and I couldn't see one thing on strokes in the waiting room and I called the doctor over and I said: "Can you tell me why there isn't any information on stroke victims in there in different languages?" '*

Attitudes towards others with aphasia

Alf's approach towards other people who have aphasia is to take their part and to try to work together with them. He has developed a strong sense of the collective identity of aphasic people and tries to develop that ethos. Struggling to educate others about his own aphasia, he has become aware both of the vulnerability and the rights of people who have aphasia. With other members of the self-help group, Alf identifies and tries to break down the barriers encountered by people who have a communication impairment.

But Alf's response to others with aphasia is not typical. Aphasic people may not always bring positive, supportive feelings to encounters with others. Meeting others who are in the same situation can trigger a range of feelings, from delight and relief to fear and rejection. Some people feel distressed when they are expected to mix with others who are very different from themselves, despite the fact that they, too, have aphasia. Some people misunderstand the meanings of others and misinterpret the difficulties they face. Some people simply do not like being in a group. Sometimes identifying with others is too difficult and painful. Attitudes to others with aphasia can be very complex.

Different ways of seeing others with aphasia

- *'They need to be pushed on. Push push push.'*
- *'Some of them are worse off than me. I feel very sorry for them.'*
- *'Now I am able to say something, I don't want it to put me back down.'*
- *'I suppose I do it because I have to enjoy it. — If I was normal it wouldn't be my cup of tea.'*
- *'There's a stroke club and I went in and there's all old people . . . all in wheelchairs and I thought: "I don't . . . don't want to go."'*
- *'You're all dealing with it, all encouraging each other.'*
- *'Just normal. They're just normal people aren't they?'*
- *'He could speak if he wanted to. But he didn't want to.'*

'Too much of with me disabled': personal identity and aphasia

Part of the process of adapting to impairments which are suddenly acquired and long-lasting seems to involve developing a new sense of self, or personal identity, which takes on the new situation. For many, this is a long drawn out and difficult process.

Although **Madge's** support system has helped her to cope in practical terms with her marked physical impairment, she has difficulty adapting her identity or sense of self to her new situation. Although she is comfortable in environments where she is not known, she refuses to go out where she might be recognised. She expresses a sense of shame about her physical impairment and is reluctant to let anyone who knew her before her stroke see her in the wheelchair which she now uses all the time: *'I still get terrified joining in with people I know. That I will not go . . . go outside in the wheelchair. And it is the wheelchair. — I will not be pushed from the house down the road. It would upset me. I can't help it, but it's inevitable.'* While Madge avoids contact with those who knew her, she also has to face the negative attitudes of those who meet her for the first time. However, she is able to counter this and to react assertively: *' "Does she like fish?" or "Is she an old-age pensioner?" Asking my daughter-in-law and I answer. I say: "I'm not going to sit here and let this go on." — Looking at me like I'd not only had a stroke, I was a little bit mentally ill as well.'* Madge's account reveals the sense of stigma which she associates with her visible, physical impairment and with the symbol of her wheelchair. This springs partly from her own feelings about disability and partly from the attitudes of those around her. The prejudices she encounters confirm her feelings that her impairment is something shameful. One of the ways in which she deals with this is to keep away from her old stamping-grounds, her pub, her bingo club, her street. She keeps a physical distance from environments in which her new self and her old self might be compared. In the safety of her own home, and in environments where she is not known, she has developed both practical ways of coping and a more confident sense of her new self.

Aphasic people who have no marked physical or sensory impairments have to try and deal with much less tangible evidence of disability. They, too, have to start the process of reconstructing a new identity, but can be uncertain about the nature of what has happened, especially because it is not visible. Like others who have invisible impairments, many decide to try and keep it hidden.

Following her stroke, **Jenny** wished to return to work as a school cleaner, but was unable to do so because of her right-sided weakness. Taking stock of her physical difficulties, which have now receded, she remembers her surprise when she found herself bracketed with those who have a disability: *'Even my own daughter . . . I said to her I'd* *like to go back to work . . . she said: "No. You're not able to go back to work. Full stop. That's it. Get that in your head. You're disabled."'* Jenny had some difficulties claiming benefits and thinks this may have been due to the fact that both her physical and language impairments were not obvious: *'I didn't know you could claim anything because nobody ever told you anything. — I suppose that's my attitude. They should tell me. Perhaps they don't think I'm ill enough.'* Jenny understands why it is difficult for others to know she has a language impairment: *'I thought a stroke was . . . you could see that somebody's had a stroke. I didn't realise that you could never tell. — I'm normal . . . well, look normal. But people with strokes are not normal. — I think a lot of people wouldn't believe you because to look at me it doesn't look as if you had a stroke. — People don't know what to think.'* Jenny points out that her aphasia is even less apparent than most, because it affects her ability to understand what is being said rather than causing her any noticeable difficulty with speaking. Because she finds it difficult to recognise when things are going wrong, Jenny finds herself reluctant to call attention to her aphasia: *'I wouldn't go and say: "I've had a stroke, you know, I can't understand" because they were talking to me and sometimes I didn't even know. — I've often, when people are talking to me, gone into a . . . I call it a haze but it's not really. It's just I'm looking at them but I don't know what they're saying to me. Often my daughter said: "Oh you're far away . . . what you thinking about?" I'm not really. I'm really thinking about what they're saying to me. You know, it's to cotton on to it. I think that was more because I didn't want anybody to know that there's something wrong.'*

'Sorry, I'm aphasic'. 'You're what?': keeping aphasia hidden

Jenny's account suggests that one of the reasons people keep their aphasia hidden may be the uncertain, intangible nature which makes it difficult to understand and to explain. Drawing attention to aphasia might place an unwelcome burden of having to explain it upon the aphasic person. Not only is this process a struggle, but it can be costly.

For *Alf*, making phone calls to enquire about social services has proved an expensive business: *'I keep on saying to myself that I'm going to keep quiet . . . not say I'm aphasic, because the majority of the public does not know what the meaning is . . . because I have to explain to them what is aphasic. — "Please, I've had a stroke. I'm aphasic and have problems. Would you speak very very slow?" — And they end up me and them practically arguing on the phone to slow down and I go: "I am aphasic" and that*

> *confuses them because they haven't got a clue what aphasic is. — And then it always is: "Oh yes, my aunt had a stroke" or "My uncle had a stroke." — "Oh isn't that a shame?" I'm not even worried whether it's a shame and I go: "Oh never mind, never mind, never mind." And I come off my phone maybe three quarters of an hour after and I go: "Well why do I have to worry about this? It's costing me money on the telephone." '*

Alf becomes irritated when he encounters ignorance about aphasia. He is reluctant to reveal his aphasia, partly because of the difficulty and tedium of explaining it and partly because he feels frustrated by the responses he meets. Many share Alf's feelings and choose to hide their aphasia. Strikingly, those who do try to explain their aphasia to others generally start off by apologising.

'*I'm sorry, I'm aphasic*': apologising for aphasia

- *'The shop . . . I'm sorry a stroke. I'm sorry. Speak and help and point.'*
- *'Sort of thank you for listening, sort of thing.'*
- *'I'm very sorry, I got a speech problem.'*
- *'If you don't mind, I'm sorry. I can't talk properly.'*
- *'I'm sorry my stroke. No I'm sorry, you know. With me my stroke slow speaking . . . um talking. And thank you.'*

Some different ways of thinking about disability

The ways in which aphasic people describe their impairment reflect different, deeply held beliefs which combine both personal and societal views of disability. A brief summary shows how diverse interpretations of disability can be. For example, from one perspective, it can be seen as a personal tragedy which the individual must strive to overcome by drawing on qualities such as bravery and patience, and relying on the care and support of others. This view is often evident in the way in which disabled people are portrayed in the popular press. Inevitably, it influences the ways in which aphasic people see themselves.

Another powerful view of disability sees it in terms of the individual's inability to function 'normally' and to carry out everyday tasks. This view underpins some medical and therapeutic approaches to disability. Restoring a degree of 'normal function' is often the aim of therapy. In the United Kingdom, this way of defining disability is also used as a basis for administrative decisions regarding a person's capacity for work and eligibility for financial support.

However, such ways of thinking about disability have not gone unchallenged. In recent years, groups of disabled people have got together to redefine disability in terms which have nothing to do with ideas of cure and care. From this perspective, disability is seen not in terms of individual limitations and inabilities. Rather, it is felt to be caused by different sorts of *barriers and obstacles* faced by those who have impairments. Seen in this way, if the barriers are removed, the disability ceases to exist. Thus a person who uses a wheelchair is disabled not by being unable to walk, but by the fact that the doorway is not wide enough or it is only possible to get into a building using stairs.

This view has developed from the concerns of those who have physical and sensory impairments, and has drawn on some of the principles underpinning feminist and civil rights campaigns. It poses a challenge to traditional medical, administrative and charitable views of disability. It also challenges the aims of rehabilitation and therapy. From this point of view, rehabilitation should be concerned with the identification and removal of barriers, rather than the improvement of the individual's abilities.

How far do the views of aphasic people themselves fit with these different ways of thinking about disability?

'I can't speak what I want to speak': **the restrictions imposed by aphasia**

People who have aphasia are only too well aware of their difficulties with communication and their inabilities. The limitations make themselves felt in every aspect of daily life. Aphasia can affect every task, every function which involves communication in domestic, family, work, leisure and social life. Making and receiving phone calls, writing letters, joining in conversations, dealing with tax and personal finances, making notes, discussing a medical problem, following a talk or lecture, listening to the radio, leaving a message for someone, giving directions, finding the right change — the list of frustrations and limitations is never-ending.

If disability is defined as the extent to which an individual is limited in ability to carry out everyday tasks and functions then people who have aphasia are clearly disabled by their communication impairment. Despite this, aphasia seems to have been disregarded in the development of the administrative categories which determine whether or not someone is capable of working or is eligible for Incapacity Benefit. In 'The all work test' the person's physical capacity for work is largely judged on ability to carry out everyday tasks such as carrying 2.5 kg of potatoes, or turning the control knobs on a cooker. Communication impairments fall within this 'physical disabilities' section, and are defined simply in terms of trouble with making oneself understood, and hearing problems.

While difficulty making oneself understood might be one manifestation of aphasia, it also affects many other aspects of communication, for example, understanding others, writing, and reading. Hearing is not affected by aphasia. Similarly, aphasia does not seem to fit comfortably within the 'mental disabilities' section, in which 'difficulty concentrating on a magazine article' (which might, superficially, describe an aphasic person's problem) is bracketed with descriptions of behaviours characteristic of illnesses such as depression and alcoholism. It seems that those who construct such categorisations, while they might be aware of many physical, sensory and mental impairments, have little knowledge of language impairment.

'The radio blaring. The pub bloody blaring': the barriers facing people with aphasia

Aphasia can be seen as a disability in terms of the limitations it imposes. But how does it fit with the definitions made by disabled people, which are concerned not with the limitations of the individual, but with the barriers they face? In some ways, it is easy to appreciate the barriers encountered by people with physical and sensory impairments — the narrow doorways, the high roadside kerbs, the lack of ramps, the inaccessible public transport. But to what extent do people who have aphasia encounter environmental barriers? How far is their access to communication blocked, and by what?

The most obvious barrier to communication is clearly a part of the physical environment. Noise of any kind can often interfere with the aphasic person's access to communication making it difficult to follow what is said and to contribute. Sources of noise include TV, radio, background music, tannoy announcements, washing machines, fans, roadworks, chatter and laughter. People handle the noise problem in different ways. Some make a case for background noise to be reduced so that they can take part in what is going on. Others simply remove themselves from noisy situations and look for quiet environments. For the aphasic person, noise is the most obvious equivalent of inaccessible buildings. This barrier is one which is faced by many other people with different types of impairment, such as deafness.

Other parallels with the concerns of those who have physical and sensory impairments can be found in the provision of appropriate aids and appliances. Those who are unable to walk need proper access to buildings which will accommodate a wheelchair. They benefit from having the best possible design of chair to suit their needs. Some aphasic people benefit from using appliances to support their communication, such as word-processors, spell-checkers, appropriate software, answerphones and alarm systems. Items like these can support the aphasic person's access to communication.

But it is important not to be too literal and concrete when thinking about barriers. The person with aphasia has to function in a physical environment, but also in a language environment. The language environment is the written and spoken language which surrounds the aphasic person. This may be too fast, too complex, too abstract to be understood. Those communicating with aphasic people may not place enough emphasis on checking out what is helpful and what has been understood. Thus, the very way in which a conversation is conducted can obstruct the person with aphasia.

Sharon's social life changed abruptly with the onset of her aphasia. Visits to theatres, pubs and clubs and attendance at evening classes became difficult, partly because of the noisy environment which blocked her attempts to join in with conversations and discussions: *'In the pub lots of people laughing and joking and speaking out and "What?" "Excuse me?" Rely all the time maybe quiet in the park or maybe one to one is alright. No it's . . . in the pub is no fun. And all the time classes, maybe one to one is alright maybe think about the teacher visiting here one hour one hour — one to one reading and writing. But the money — no forget it.'* Sharon has become adept at stating what her requirements are, for example, when making phone calls to the council. However, she still becomes aggravated by some of the responses she meets: *'Well on the phone I said: "I'm sorry my stroke and slowly speaking . . . um . . . talking slow." Once or twice "What?" "I'm sorry, I'm sorry my stroke . . ." Angry and slam the phone down.'* Sharon finds that she reacts angrily to friends and acquaintances who talk in her company as if she is not there, who patronise her, or who appear to think she has regressed to childhood: *'Maybe man or woman with me . . . the infant, or is dumb with me. — Yes, I'm sorry. Me and myself on my own or the adult and normal with me.'*

Sharon's account shows how she is facing a number of different kinds of barriers. She encounters noise, distraction, and language which is too fast for her to understand. But she also encounters other barriers in the form of other people's attitudes towards her. She knows, too, that she will be unable to continue her education, unless she can pay for special help. Her opportunities are restricted.

Sharon's account is not unusual. Although most aphasic people do not use the term 'barriers', they do talk, in detail, about things which get in their way and which prevent them from doing what they want to do.

Far from locating these limitations entirely within themselves, they point out that, if the obstacles were removed, they would be able to move on.

The disabling barriers encountered by aphasic people can be classified into four main groups. Some barriers spring up from the physical and language environment. Structural barriers arise when systems, services, opportunities and resources are inappropriate, inadequate or simply not available. Examples of structural barriers might include the lack of a counselling service, minimal access to social services, lack of flexibility in teaching methods and inappropriate special educational needs support. Access to work may be restricted, for example because lengthy, rapidly run meetings are not adapted to meet the aphasic person's needs. Attitudinal barriers arise from the responses of other people, which can range from pity to prejudice. Informational barriers spring up when people with aphasia cannot find the information they need or it is presented in such a way that it cannot be understood.

Disabling barriers encountered by people with aphasia

- **Environmental barriers (physical and language environment):**
  'People talking all at once . . . the noise . . . I can't cope with that.'
  'I go please, please, please slow down.'
  'Everything's in a hurry.'
  'Simple word, not big word. And capital letters.'
  'They ask you complicated questions.'

- **Structural barriers (resources, opportunities, services and support):**
  'There should be a counsellor of some sort, shouldn't there?'
  'Obviously for meetings for me to express myself is pretty difficult . . .'
  'Social service, forget it.'
  'I think: "Well, why nobody to help me? Why? Why?"'

- **Attitudinal barriers:**
  'When I go to a restaurant or a pub, I get ignored totally.'
  'The people sees . . . they do not give damn.'
  'Some of them actually thought I think you are an imbecile.'
  'They assume you're deaf or something like that.'
  'They couldn't understand what's wrong with me.'
  'They don't want to know really. They got a job and that's all they care about.'

• **Informational barriers**:
  'You cannot always ask.'
  'Why, what, how?'
  'Are there social services?'
  'If they realise you don't know nothing, they don't tell you a thing.'

The experiences of the aphasic people who took part in this study clearly show how, at every turn, they encounter disabling barriers which get in their way. They also talk about how such barriers can be lifted: the teacher who gives handouts instead of expecting students to take notes, the doctor who gives time and thought to a consultation with an aphasic patient, the leaflet which is clearly and simply laid out, the social worker who checks out the best way to communicate.

How can the disabling barriers facing people with aphasia be removed?

• **Environmental barriers**
  Educate and inform non-aphasic people (including those who provide health, social care and voluntary services) so that they:

  1 Become aware of the need to develop aphasia-friendly environments.
  2 Change their spoken and written language to meet the needs of people with aphasia.
  3 Give time to encounters with aphasic people.

'Ordinary people have got to be educated all the same . . . to make them aware of what to expect from people like me.'

• **Structural barriers**
  Educate and inform those providing and organising services so that they:

  1 Become aware of the changing needs and requirements of aphasic people.
  2 Establish appropriate and adequate services and resources to meet those needs.
  3 Become accountable to people with aphasia.
  4 Develop communicative access to opportunities in work and education, for example re-structuring meetings, making agendae and minutes easier to understand, finding alternatives to note-taking.

'I think that you should actually decide that maybe three months or six months or a year or maybe two years that should be a review and so that people should actually be given hope.'

- **Attitudinal barriers**
  1 Educate and inform non-aphasic people (including those providing health, social care and voluntary services) about the nature and impact of aphasia.
  2 Challenge negative, patronising and prejudiced attitudes.
  3 Promote awareness of the barriers faced by people who have aphasia.

'Some people like doesn't mind. Other people don't want to know. They're frightened, I think they're frightened that it may happen to them. I think that's what it is. It's like cancer, cancer. A lot of people are frightened of cancer because they think of other people, they think it might be theirs as well. — You're talking to them and they want to go away. They don't want to stay and talk to you. — I don't take any notice now. If they seem to be . . . they don't understand I just tell 'em what's happened and then it's not too bad. I say: "I can't talk. I got . . . I had a stroke. You slow down." '

- **Informational barriers**
  Educate those providing information so that they:

  1 Develop understanding of the nature and impact of aphasia.
  2 Understand that the information needs of aphasic people change over time.
  3 Modify the ways in which information is presented so that it is accessible.
  4 Present information in different ways and in different languages.

'All the information should be collated in one package.'

People who took part in this study have clear ideas about how the obstacles they face could be removed, largely through a process of educating others about aphasia. However, some feel that the task of challenging and educating others is beyond them, because it requires them to use the language which has been damaged by their impairment. A commonly expressed view is that other people, including health and social care professionals, are simply not interested in learning about what aphasia really means. They do not want to know. In addition, many aphasic people take a deeply pessimistic view of the political and economic forces which block the way of any possible developments:

'The Tory Govern is not much money. Not to finish but is sorry, is no can do. See you later, sort of thing. And then another stroke victim is in offering sort of thing.'

Stephen

'It's cut down. Cut down. Cut this out. Cut this out.'

Fred

Considering aphasia from the point of view of the limitations it imposes, and from the point of view of the barriers which spring up it is possible to see how these two ways of seeing disability have very different meanings and implications. The same problem can be seen in entirely different lights according to which standpoint is taken. Thus, one person who struggles to communicate with their GP may feel it is their own fault: they have not worked hard enough at improving their language and are failing to overcome their difficulties. Another aphasic person in the same situation may feel angry with the GP for not giving enough time to the consultation or for not finding out how to support their communication.

Thinking in terms of disabling barriers helps to put a different perspective on the difficulties faced by people who have aphasia. If the problems are seen in a different way, new solutions become apparent. But some aspects of aphasia simply cannot be seen in terms of barriers. For example, what obstacle could have been removed to enable Fred to carry out his wish of making a speech at his daughter's wedding? Fred dealt with this by asking his brother-in-law to make the speech on his behalf, but this does not take away from the fact that he wanted to undertake this highly personal and symbolic task himself. Other examples of difficulties which cannot be understood in terms of barriers are listed in the box below.

Problems faced by aphasic people which cannot be understood in terms of barriers

People who have aphasia describe:

- Feeling unable to write a personal and private letter to a relative or friend.
- Feeling unable to discuss a daughter's drug addiction with the family GP in sufficient depth and detail.
- Feeling unable to talk with a son who is being bullied at school, to say the right things to console him, to make useful suggestions and to discuss the problem with a teacher.
- Feeling unable to concentrate and focus on one topic.
- Feeling unable to settle down with a book.
- Feeling unable to offer verbal comfort to a distressed partner or friend.

- Having to wait for others to help with writing a cheque in their own time.
- Missing out on gossip.
- Feeling unable to make enquiries or complaints in person.
- Being unable to have any secrets, for example because help is needed to buy birthday presents.
- Being unable to deal with daily harassment from a neighbour.
- Being unable to make a joke or put a humorous slant on a conversation.
- Losing the traces and details of a discussion or conversation.

Difficulties such as these might, at first sight, seem insignificant or trivial perhaps because they do not concern the transmission of important information or the basic communication of needs, requirements and emotions. But they indicate how aphasia can wipe out the nuances and subtleties of communication and much of the intrinsic enjoyment of using language. More importantly, they show how loss of language can lead to a damaging loss of control over the maintenance of relationships and the balance of conversations, the organisation of personal time, and over the help and support which is offered by others. Some aphasic people comment that the loss of language has rendered them powerless. They are disabled by the very nature of their aphasia.

'I wouldn't fit': aphasia and the disability movement

People who have aphasia share a number of concerns in common with other disabled people. These include a sense of exclusion, the ambiguity of sometimes invisible impairments, a desire to work towards the removal of barriers and obstacles, and a sense of scepticism about how much change is really possible through education and awareness-raising. In recent years, members of the disability movement within the United Kingdom have shown the importance of joining with others and developing a strong collective identity. Although there are often conflicts and disagreements within the movement, many people, even those who have very different impairments, actively support each other. Together, they are identifying the obstacles they face in common and starting the work of breaking them down.

Yet, despite the fact that they share this common ground, it is rare for aphasic people and other disabled people to join together in addressing common concerns. Aphasic people express the sense that they 'don't fit' with the disability movement and indeed that their aphasia is poorly understood. One reason for this may be that developments within the movement have come about largely through the efforts of disabled people who are able to use language to demand, discuss, campaign, debate and object. The issues have been defined and the challenges stated in meetings, interviews, essays, books, papers and articles. All of these depend upon written and spoken language which is often abstract and complex. This means that theories and campaigns relating to disability have been largely inaccessible to people who have language impairment. The language of the disability debate has perhaps become another barrier, reinforcing the isolation of people who have aphasia:

'The language difficulty is the most disability of all.'

Kiran

9

'I'm fed up of saying I'm sorry': learning to live with aphasia

The accounts in this study document not only the difficulties and struggles but also the endeavour of learning to live with aphasia. People who have aphasia talk about the ways in which they cope with the loss of language, the strategies they use and how they make sense of what has happened. Drawing together these diverse accounts, it is possible to discern a number of underpinning principles. These are not explicitly stated, but are embedded and entwined in the different experiences described. This final chapter seeks to draw out some of these principles, in the hope that they might be helpful to others who are suddenly confronted with loss of language.

Learning to live with aphasia

- Work towards understanding what aphasia is and the needs and requirements it imposes.

  'Language is what makes the world as it is. — If my arm was missing or my leg was, I know that my arm or leg was missing and I would grieve about that. But when it's your world . . . your sense of the world.'

- Try to find others who are in the same situation and work with them to develop a collective identity.

  'Let's be honest about it and let's all deal with it and try to help each other as much as we can.'

- Work together to identify and dismantle barriers and obstacles.

> 'We all got together. We said we're all agreed that in the beginning people talked to the person who was pushing the wheelchair, not to us. 'I suppose we all feel angry'.

- Develop a strong, aphasic, personal identity.

> 'I have had to fight for that self-respect. That I'm fed up of saying I'm sorry, I'm sorry. I do not want to say that any more. I'm _not_ sorry.'

- Expect others to share responsibility for these processes.

> 'I want to change my life in a society that has responsibility for me and I have a responsibility to it.'

Understanding the nature of aphasia and the needs and requirements it imposes

Many aphasic people stress the importance of understanding and acknowledging major significance of what has happened to their language. This means getting to know the aphasia, and the demands which it imposes. It seems important to understand the cause and the nature of aphasia and what the outlook is. This process can take many years, as the aphasic person goes through experiences which highlight different aspects of aphasia, comes to understand what can and cannot be done, and learns what support is required.

'Speech is alright most of the time but it does go when I'm tired or stressful situations. I can read most things but after ten minutes I can see it but I can't understand what I'm reading. — I could read bits and pieces, but I could never read the whole book. I would get far too tired. The coursework we used to have two or three weeks to do an essay, so that weren't too bad. I could do it half an hour at a time. I couldn't do it all in one go. You had to discipline yourself to sit down for half an hour and have a good crack at it.'

Trevor

Finding others and developing a collective identity

Many aphasic people stress the importance of contact with others who are in the same situation. The rewarding nature of meeting others who are 'in the same boat' makes itself felt in every context, even those which emphasise treatment, cure and care. Aphasia can make people feel isolated and excluded. Aphasic people need opportunities to meet others in a variety of contexts.

*'When I looked at them . . . there was . . . We can understand each other, quite
simply. That we are on the same boat. — The important thing was . . . you didn't
have to say a word. It was brilliant. I don't know why I felt so wonderful . . . I
suppose it's because of that. I know that she . . . he were the same as me.'*

Kiran

Identifying and dismantling barriers

Some aphasic people are confronting the shame they feel about their language impairment. They are questioning how far they should blame
themselves when things go wrong in their interactions with others. This
means thinking about the problems which arise in everyday life and
trying to work out what the barriers are and how they might be lifted.
Could someone talk more slowly? Could something be written more
simply or laid out more clearly? Learning to see aphasia in this way means
that the aphasic person tackles problems by looking outwards rather than
inwards.

*'If they seem to be they don't understand I just tell them what's happened and
then it's not too bad. — I had a stroke. You talk slow. Slow down, because if
somebody's talking I don't always hear the first words.'*

Rob

*'It's educating them into a different way of thought. That just because someone is
incapacitated in that nature doesn't mean that they're any less intelligent or
incapable.'*

Rebecca

Developing a strong aphasic, personal identity

This refers to the 'inside work' which the aphasic person undertakes in
constructing a new sense of self. It means understanding the limitations
imposed by aphasia but also acknowledging personal strengths and assets.
People come to think of themselves as having aphasia, but also having a
lot to offer. For some, it is no longer necessary to apologise.

*'It's confidence, it's all about confidence. — When I first . . . embarrassed about
everything you know. — Perhaps the years seem to have gone by and my aphasia
. . . I mean I am still aphasic, obviously, but it doesn't seem to matter any more.
My loss isn't so great anymore. So if I miss a few words it doesn't really matter
anymore. — I'm one of the world's listeners now. I'm not one of the talkers.'*

Judith

Expecting others to share the responsibility

The accounts given in this study show the central importance of sharing the concerns and responsibilities brought by aphasia with other people. They detail the stigma and isolation which can occur when a person with aphasia only looks inward to find explanations and solutions. Those aphasic people who have found allies and advocates have done so by drawing on a number of different personal resources including honesty and assertiveness. The special nature of aphasia means this is not easy or straightforward. The process can be eased when non-aphasic people approach those who have aphasia proactively, thinking in terms of respect, rights and fairness rather than cure and care:

'Nobody will ever help you unless you ask. If you cannot ask, which is true — you cannot always ask — you may not be able to speak, so you're in limbo-land. There must be a friend somewhere. You must have a friend somewhere on this earth. You cannot be on your own complete.'

Alf

Of course, many people experience profound feelings of sadness, anger and regret about their aphasia and sometimes these feelings can obstruct their progress. But the accounts given in this study also show that it is possible to find some personal gains in the experience of losing language. This can happen in a number of different ways. For example, aphasia can become the stimulus for taking new directions in work and study. Some find that having aphasia allows them more opportunity to concentrate on the things they enjoy and which are really important to them, such as personal relationships. Some find that their aphasia opens up their lives, allowing the opportunity to develop new skills and bringing them into contact with people they would never otherwise have met.

While it is possible to list such gains and benefits, there is a danger that these might be viewed simplistically as ways in which a person can 'come to terms' or 'make the best' of aphasia. It is perhaps tempting to stress the heroic qualities of people who develop a positive view of their aphasia, and to see them as in some way having 'overcome' their difficulties. But there is no getting away from the fact that life with aphasia is a daily struggle. Aphasic people find that they can no longer make predictions based on previous knowledge and experience. They are precipitated into an uncertain and often hostile world, in which every encounter exposes their fragility and forces them to face and redefine their sense of self. They can feel isolated, vulnerable, excluded and powerless. But in some ways, the experience of aphasia, harsh and unrelenting as it is, offers the chance to make a new start. Aphasic people are given the opportunity to look inwards and face themselves as they are, without language, and with all the trappings and busy-ness of pre-aphasic life stripped away. Seen from this perspective, it is possible for aphasia to become not an end, but a beginning.

'It's a starting all over. New life, really.'

Appendix:
About the project

The background to the project

The Aphasia and Disability Project ran from March 1994 to September 1996. The project was funded by the Joseph Rowntree Foundation. It was carried out by the Department of Clinical Communication Studies, City University, London, UK. The research team comprised two aphasic people and two speech and language therapists who joined forces to design, carry out and disseminate the project. They were supported throughout by the input of two advisory panels, one consisting of people who have aphasia and one made up of academic, clinical and professional specialists. Both panels provided suggestions, feedback and advice at regular intervals through the course of the project. A consultant provided guidance and training in the use of qualitative research methods, and monitored the analysis of the project data.

The idea for the project sprang from three main sources. Current trends in the sociology of illness formed one major influence. These highlighted the importance of seeking to understand the 'insider' account of chronic conditions, rather than maintaining the professional perspective. Another influence derived from developments in the disability discourse, which suggested new ways of thinking about the causes and nature of disability and promoted reflection on the process and principles of research. Thirdly, despite the fact that aphasia had been extensively studied, it was clear that the experience of living with aphasia in the long term was poorly understood. Given these influences, the project was designed with two main aims in mind. First, it aimed to explore the long-term effects of aphasia, both in terms of its impact upon people's lives and in terms of how it is perceived and understood by the people who have it. Secondly, the project aimed to investigate the disabling nature of aphasia.

The methodology used in the project

Given the aims and ethos of the project, it was decided that qualitative methodology was the most appropriate for the task of exploring the long-term consequences and significance of aphasia. In-depth interviewing is one qualitative method which explores the experiences, views and perspectives of the people whom the research is about. Despite the difficulties which seemed likely to beset the task of interviewing people who have a communication impairment, it was felt that this method was the most suitable for the purpose of the study as it offered the best means of getting 'inside' the experience of aphasia. In-depth interviewing allows important topics and issues to be raised by the respondent, in addition to those broached by the researcher. It offers the chance for in-depth exploration of such issues, in the terms and language of the people taking part. Its flexibility means that people who have communication difficulties, who might struggle to respond to standard questioning, have the opportunity to describe their experience and express their views and concerns in their own way. However, the flexibility of the method does not mean that it is unsystematic. This project was planned to be methodologically robust and rigorous at every stage – in design, sampling, implementation and analysis.

The respondents

In order to ensure that the long-term impact was described, it was decided that the sample should be confined to people who had at least five years' experience of aphasia. In the event, two respondents were slightly under this limit. One respondent had been aphasic for 18 years, but was able to recall the experience of stroke and the onset of aphasia in minute and vivid detail. It was also decided to exclude people who had become aphasic as a result of an event other than a stroke (for example, head injury or progressive neurological condition) and those living in care settings.

Once these criteria were decided, the respondents were selected through three sources: hospital records; speech and language therapy records; and the records of voluntary and charitable associations. Ethical approval for the project was gained in each health district or trust before information was sent out to potential participants. Those who indicated their willingness to take part were then contacted by phone or letter and an appointment was arranged. In most cases, respondents were interviewed at home.

Fifty aphasic people took part in the project. They were purposively selected to ensure that a range of characteristics and circumstances was represented. These were as follows:

Gender
The sample comprised 21 women and 29 men.

Age
The sample was selected to ensure that the experience of young and elderly aphasic people was represented. The youngest respondent was 26 years old and the oldest 92 years old. The age distribution was as follows:

Number of respondents in each age band
under 45 years: 8
46 54 years: 21
65–74 years: 16
75 years and above: 5

Severity of aphasia
One-third of the sample was made up of people with severe or marked aphasia which significantly affected their ability to take part in a conversation. They were invited to take part in the project because it was felt that their experience was important and they should not be excluded. These interviews were particularly challenging, and required the interviewers to modify their questioning and to encourage different forms of communication. Obviously, if a person had severe comprehension problems sometimes it was not possible to continue. However, it was often difficult to tell in advance whether or not a person would be able to participate. This was judged by the interviewers on each occasion by a number of exploratory remarks and questions. The remainder of the sample comprised people whose aphasia was less severe.

Living circumstances
Approximately one-third of participants were living on their own. The remainder were living with their families.

Physical impairment
Approximately half the respondents had some severe physical impairment as a result of their stroke, in addition to aphasia.

Location
Respondents were selected from different urban and rural locations throughout the UK.

Ethnicity
Respondents were sampled to ensure that the experience of people from different ethnic groups was represented.

The topic guide

The topic guide was designed to ensure that certain issues were systematically covered in the interviews. Although they followed the topic guide, the interviewers were encouraged to be flexible in tuning in to the communicative needs and abilities of each respondent.

The topic guide covered a number of issues:

• Personal and household information.
• The pattern of daily activities and occupations.
• The experience of having a stroke.
• First perceptions of aphasia.
• The impact of aphasia upon work, education, finances, leisure pursuits and personal relationships.
• The experience and evaluation of health, social care, welfare and voluntary services.
• Information needs and access.
• Personal understanding of aphasia.
• The disabling nature of aphasia.

The researchers were offered training in in-depth interviewing and the support of a trained interviewer. Three pilot interviews were carried out.

Analysis of the interview information

Every interview was tape-recorded, with the permission of the interviewee, and then transcribed verbatim. At all points, confidentiality and anonymity were given high priority. In this book and in other forms of dissemination, names and some personal details have been changed to maintain confidentiality. Issues arising from the interviews were classified and indexed. Then the data was organised in charts or matrices which displayed individual responses, themes and issues. Subsequent analysis of the material contained in the charts indicated the range and pattern of views on each issue. This method of analysing the data from in-depth interviews is known as the 'Framework' method and has been developed by the research organisation Social and Community Planning Research (Ritchie and Spencer 1994).

References

Ritchie, J. and Spencer, L. (1994) 'Qualitative data analysis for applied policy research', in A. Bryman and R. Burgess (eds) *Analysing Qualitative Data*. London: Routledge.

Further reading

The following list of books and papers may be useful for people who wish to read further on the topics of aphasia, chronic illness and disability. The list is by no means comprehensive.

Action for Dysphasic Adults (1995) *National Directory: National Register of Language Opportunities for those with Dysphasia and their Families*. London: ADA.

Anderson, R. (1992) *The Aftermath of Stroke*. Cambridge: University Press.

Bury, M. (1991) The sociology of chronic illness: a review of research and prospects, *Sociology of Health and Illness*, 13(4): 452–68.

Disability Alliance (1995) *Disability Rights Handbook*. London: Disability Alliance Educational and Research Associations.

Edelman, G. and Greenwood, R. (eds) (1992) *Jumbly Words and Rights where Wrongs should be: the Experience of Aphasia from the Inside*. Kibworth: Far Communications.

French, S. (1994) (ed.) *On Equal Terms: Working with Disabled People*. Oxford: Butterworth-Heinemann.

Hales, G. (1996) (ed.) *Beyond Disability – Towards an Enabling Society*. London: Sage.

Holland, A. and Forbes, M. (eds) (1993) *Aphasia Treatment: World Perspectives*. London: Chapman and Hall.

Jordan, L. and Kaiser, W. (1996) *Aphasia – a Social Approach*. London: Chapman and Hall.

Kagan, A. and Gailey, G. (1993) Functional is not enough: training of conversation partners for aphasic adults, in A. Holland and M. Forbes (eds) *Aphasia Treatment: World Perspectives*. London: Chapman and Hall.

King's Fund Forum on Stroke (1988) *The Treatment of Stroke: Consensus Statement*. London: King Edward's Hospital Fund for London.

Kleinman, A. (1988) *The Illness Narratives*. Harvard: Basic Books.

Lisle, R. (1996) *When Granny Couldn't Speak*. London: ADA.

Marshall, J. and Carlson, E. (1993) *How to Help the Dysphasic Person*, series. London: ADA.

Stroke Association Community Services (1993) *Dysphasic Support*. London: The Stroke Association.

Swain, J., Finkelstein, V., French, S. and Oliver, M. (eds) (1993) *Disabling Barriers, Enabling Environments*. London: Sage.

WITH THIS BODY
CARING AND DISABILITY IN MARRIAGE

Gillian Parker

This book breaks new ground by examining the views both of younger people who become disabled after marriage and of their partners who become involved in helping and supporting them. It explores the giving and receiving of personal care in marriage, and the roles of informal networks, services and income in supporting these couples and their children. It shows how, in the absence of help and support from elsewhere, couples are left in an extremely precarious position – practically, financially, emotionally, and socially. Disabled people argue the need for resources and services that would allow them to be independent of 'informal' help. This book shows that age, class, gender and existing power relations in the marriage affect the experience of both disability and caring and the extent to which 'independence' from informal help is seen by either partner as a legitimate or desirable goal.

Contents
The invisible marriage: disability and caring – Negotiating the boundaries: physical and personal care in marriage – 'They've got their own lives to lead': the role of informal networks – Help from formal services – The economic effect of caring and disability – Disability, caring and marriage – Children, disability and caring – It hurts more inside: being a spouse carer – Conclusions – Appendix – References – Index.

160pp   0 335 09946 7 (Paperback)   0 335 09947 5 (Hardback)

CARING FOR PEOPLE
HELP AT THE FRONTLINE

Jenny Rogers

A careworker is in the 'frontline'; is often the person who deals first with clients who are frightened, confused, angry and lonely; who washes, toilets and dresses clients; who sits with a dying client and deals with the bereaved relatives. *Caring for People* provides invaluable and practical guidance for all frontline carers. It discusses how best to empathise with the client, how to listen, assess risks, encourage clients' self esteem and independence. It deals with the routine daily tasks, and how to cope with the emergencies. It shows how to avoid stress in the job, and advises on career development. It is a down to earth handbook for all careworkers.

Contents
Introduction – The need for care – being a client – The fundamentals of caring – Helping with daily living – Listening and talking – Dealing with emergencies – Death and bereavement – Looking after yourself – Making progress – Booklist – Index.

176pp   0 335 09429 5 (Paperback)   0 335 09430 9 (Hardback)